GASTRIC BYPASS COOKBOOK

Top 100 Delicious and Healthy Recipes for Lunch, Salads, and Smoothies

STEPHANIE LEWIS

© **Copyright 2022 - All rights reserved.**

The content contained within this book may not be reproduced, duplicated, or transmitted without direct written permission from the author or the publisher.

Under no circumstances will any blame or legal responsibility be held against the publisher, or author, for any damages, reparation, or monetary loss due to the information contained within this book, either directly or indirectly.

Legal Notice:

This book is copyright protected. It is only for personal use. You cannot amend, distribute, sell, use, quote or paraphrase any part, or the content within this book, without the consent of the author or publisher.

Disclaimer Notice:

Please note the information contained within this document is for educational and entertainment purposes only. All effort has been executed to present accurate, up to date, reliable, complete information. No warranties of any kind are declared or implied. Readers acknowledge that the author is not engaging in the rendering of legal, financial, medical, or professional advice. The content within this book has been derived from various sources. Please consult a licensed professional before attempting any techniques outlined in this book.

By reading this document, the reader agrees that under no circumstances is the author responsible for any losses, direct or indirect, that are incurred as a result of the use of information contained within this document, including, but not limited to, errors, omissions, or inaccuracies.

Table of Contents

Introduction 1

Chapter One: Gastric Bypass Diet and Nutrition 3
    Stages of Recovery 4

Chapter Two: What to Eat 7
    Dietary Suggestions for Stage 1 8
    Dietary Suggestions for Stage 2 8
    Dietary Suggestions for Stage 3 8
    Dietary Suggestions for Stage 4 9
    What to Avoid 9

Chapter Three: Tips to Remember 13

Chapter Four: The Road to Recovery and Better Health 17
    Tips to a Speedy Recovery 17
    Tips for Successful Meal Planning 23

Chapter Five: Gastric Bypass Smoothie Recipes 29
    Banana Cream Protein Shake 30
    Avocado Smoothie 31
    Berry Oatmeal Smoothie 32
    Gingerbread Smoothie 33
    Powerhouse Smoothie 34

Watermelon Strawberry Smoothie 36

Superfood Rainbow Smoothie... 38

Orange Lemonade Smoothie... 41

Green Cleansing Smoothie 42

Blueberry Lemonade Smoothie... 44

Carrot Smoothie 45

Berry, Banana and Kale Smoothie 46

Avocado and Papaya Smoothie... 48

Layered Banana Split Protein Smoothie................................. 50

Orange Creamsicle Smoothie 52

Pina Colada Protein Smoothie.. 53

Raspberry Watermelon Mojito Smoothie 54

Layered Smoothie Bowl... 55

Green Smoothie Protein Shake 57

Butterfinger Protein Shake 58

Chapter Six: Gastric Bypass Lunch Recipes 59

Chicken Broth 59

Creamy Shrimp Scampi Puree 62

Turkey Tacos with Refried Beans Puree 64

Chimichurri Chicken Puree 66

Sweet Potato Puree... 68

Chicken and Black Bean Mole Puree 70

Jell-O Mousse 72

Lentil, Haricot Bean and Chickpea Soup................................ 73

Curried Acorn Squash Cream Soup with Coconut Milk............ 76

Three Bean Turkey Chili.. 79

Korean Turkey Bowl	82
Creamy White Bean Soup with Kale	84
Buffalo Ranch Chicken	87
Cauliflower Soup	88
Thai Red Curry with Vegetables	90
Jeweled Rice Pilaf	93
Roasted Vegetable Pasta	95
Greek Pita Sandwiches	98
Tomato Stuffed Roasted Eggplant	102
Thai Tofu Quinoa Bowl	104
Tofu and Broccoli Quiche	107
Black Bean and Brown Rice Casserole	109
Jerk Chicken Bowl	111
Greek Chicken Burgers	113
Tabbouleh and Chicken	115
Parmesan Crusted Chicken Tenders	117
Thai Chicken Satay with Spicy Peanut Sauce	119
Chicken Cordon Bleu Wonton Cupcakes	121
Chicken Pepper Nachos	123
Mexican Chicken Quinoa Salad Wraps	125
Chicken Tetrazzini	128
Asian Chicken Lettuce Wraps	130
Mediterranean Chicken Wraps	132
Chicken Chile Verde	134
Sour Cream Chicken Enchiladas	136
Zucchini Noodles with Turkey Marinara	138
Fajita Turkey Burger	141

Moroccan Turkey Meatballs 143
Turkey Meatloaf 146
Turkey Tagine with Fruit and Nut Couscous and Yogurt Dip . 148
Ground Beef and Vegetable Stew 153
Pizza Casserole 155
Bacon Cheeseburger Casserole 157
Easy Beef Chili 160
Ancho Chile Ground Beef Tacos 163
Cheesesteak Stuffed Peppers 166
Beef Bourguignon Stew 168
Thai Coconut Fish Curry 170
Grilled Shrimp Tacos with Cilantro Lime Coconut Cream Sauce 172
Fish Taco Cabbage Bowls 175
Angel Hair Pasta with Lemon Grilled Shrimp, Spinach, and Pine Nuts 177
Smoked Salmon Sushi Bowls 179

Chapter Seven: Gastric Bypass Salad Recipes 181
Classic Pureed Tuna Salad 181
Egg Salad 183
Soft Crab Salad 184
Chicken Salad 185
Taco Salad 187
Grilled Steak with Baby Arugula and Parmesan Salad 189
Strawberry Avocado Salad with Honey Glazed Grilled Salmon 191
Sardine Salad Niçoise 193

Arugula Salad with Salmon, Avocado and Tomato 195

Herbed Shrimp with Tomato and Spinach Salad 197

Mediterranean Tuna Salad 199

Grilled Shrimp Asian Salad with Thai Peanut Dressing 201

Chicken Avocado Caprese Salad 204

Chicken Nachos Salad with Avocado Dressing 207

Buttermilk Chicken with Chopped Salad 210

Summer Strawberry and Chicken Salad with
Sweet Thyme Dressing 212

Red Quinoa, Couscous and Arugula Salad with
Sweet Pimiento Dressing 214

Summer Salad with Buttermilk Vinaigrette 217

Rainbow Salad with Za'atar Yogurt Dressing 219

Cucumber, Corn, Black Bean, and Avocado Salad 221

Thai Quinoa Salad 222

Southwestern Salad with Black Beans 224

Spiralized Apple Salad 226

Three Bean Mediterranean Salad 228

Winter Green Salad with Pomegranate Dressing 230

Summer Salad with Creamy Italian Dressing 232

Watermelon Tomato Salad 234

Orzo Salad 236

Conclusion **238**

Resources **240**

Introduction

There are several factors in life that you cannot control. One of the few and the most important things you can regulate is your health. You are the only one responsible for taking care of it; no one else can do it for you. Undergoing a gastric bypass surgery shows your commitment to improving your overall health and wellbeing. A gastric bypass is a surgical procedure through which the size of the stomach is reduced to promote weight loss. In certain cases, it is a lifesaving procedure and recommended only after all other possible options are exhausted. This surgical procedure permanently changes different aspects of your daily nutrition. From what you eat to how much you can eat, your body's ability to handle the food consumed will change. Making a few lifestyle changes and developing healthy habits is the only means to retain the benefits offered by this surgery.

After undergoing a gastric bypass, you must stick to an extremely strict diet during recovery. The diet consists of four stages that slowly recondition your stomach and digestive tract to handle food as it did before. You will be on a fully liquid diet during the first stage, whereas the second stage introduces pureed foods. During the third stage, you can reintroduce soft foods and, finally, shift to solid foods. Getting to the fourth stage can take at least 6 weeks.

Nutrition plays an extremely important role in recovery and maintaining the benefits associated with gastric bypass. You'll need to pay attention to not just the type of food you are consuming but the quantity as well. Usually, most believe that the meals they eat will be blended and extremely boring. Well, you don't have to worry about this. You also don't have to spend hours searching for gastric bypass diet-friendly recipes.

In this book, you will discover extremely delicious, easy-to-cook, and healthy lunch recipes you can consume after undergoing gastric bypass surgery. By following these recipes, you will essentially be eating your way to a healthier and fitter you. The recipes are based on the gastric bypass diet, specially designed to optimize recovery and promote weight loss and maintenance. This diet enables your body to heal from the inside and reduces the chances of complications or side effects after the surgery. Also, it is quite simple to follow once you know what to do.

So, are you excited to discover different recipes that will cater to your taste buds without compromising on nutritional needs? If yes, let us get started immediately!

Chapter One

Gastric Bypass Diet and Nutrition

Gastric bypass or Roux-en-Y gastric bypass is a surgical procedure and is typically prescribed as a weight loss remedy. In this, a small pouch is created from the stomach that directly bypasses the small intestine. After this surgical procedure, the food you eat moves from this newly created pouch and goes to the small intestine. As the name suggests, the food literally bypasses the stomach. This is also one of the most common forms of bariatric surgery. It's recommended when an individual's weight causes chronic health problems, or the said individual cannot lose weight regardless of their diet or exercise regimen. Apart from weight loss, this surgery reduces the risk of weight-related chronic health conditions such as heart diseases, type-2 diabetes, infertility, gastroesophageal reflux disease, obstructive sleep apnea, certain types of cancer, high blood pressure, and cholesterol levels.

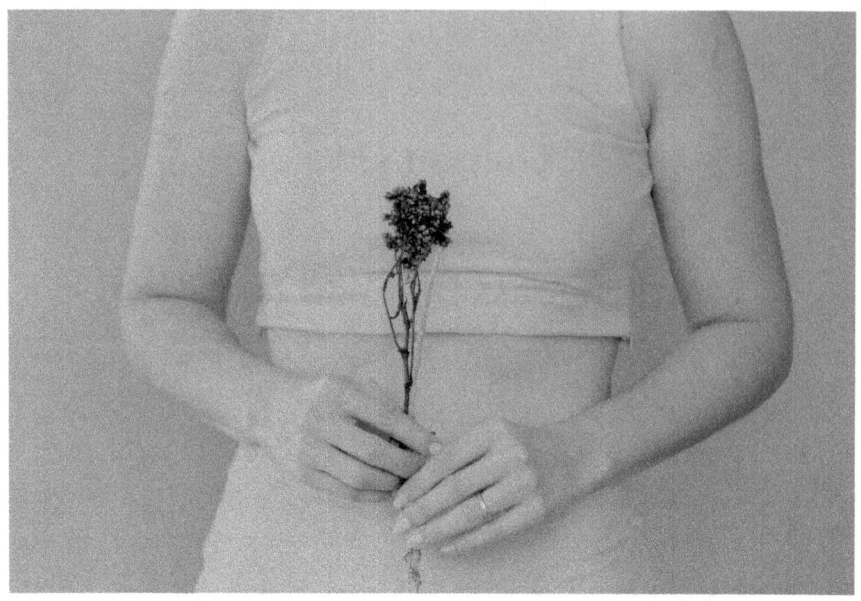

One of the most important aspects anyone who has undergone this surgery or will undergo it must remember is that it is not a silver bullet. It will not magically fix everything. Instead, think of it as the first step toward making healthy lifelong dietary changes for achieving and maintaining the ideal body weight. This procedure is rendered pointless without taking care of nutrition and diet after the surgery. Once you are armed with the right information, taking care of these things becomes extremely simple. Let's learn more about this.

Stages of Recovery

If you undergo a gastric bypass, you must make healthy dietary changes. These changes are not just needed for the time being but must become a part of your usual lifestyle. From becoming more conscious about the quality of ingredients to the portions consumed, mindful eating is needed. A typical gastric bypass diet is divided into four stages, and they are as follows.

Stage 1

The first stage consists of an entirely liquid-based diet. You must stick to a strict fluid diet for the first 12-15 days following the surgery. During this stage, the primary focus is to protect your new stomach from solid and bulky foods. The postoperative swelling in the stomach makes it even smaller than it already is. The staples in the stomach will take up to 6 weeks to be fully healed. Therefore, you cannot start eating like you used to right after the surgery. Doing this causes physical pain and increases the risk of disrupting the staples and gastric leak.

Stage 2

Once you have made it through the first two weeks and your body is responding well, you move on to the second stage of this diet. The second stage consists of pureed foods. During this stage, the primary focus is on promoting healing and reducing the risk of complications. You will need to consume only pureed foods and liquids until the fourth week after surgery. The diet you follow now will be more varied than it was in the previous stage. Full-bodied soups, stews, cooked cereals, fruits, vegetables, and sauces will now be a part of the diet.

Stage 3

You move on to the third stage of the diet after making it through the first four weeks. Internal healing will be in full swing, but your body needs longer to recover. You can gradually reintroduce different ingredients between the surgery's fourth and sixth weeks. However, you must consume only soft foods. Remember, your stomach isn't fully healed, and you must be patient. Some common foods that can be slowly reintroduced now include fish, lean meat and poultry, vegetables and fruits, legumes and rice, and some dairy products. All these foods must be extremely soft.

Stage 4

The final stage of this diet usually sets in after making it to the six-weeks mark. During this stage, swelling will be nonexistent, and the staples in the stomach will be fully healed. Solid foods can be reintroduced, but you should do it gradually. This is the time to celebrate because you have made excellent progress so far. Do not get over-excited, and do not lose patience. Instead, you need to reintroduce different solid foods slowly. Rushing into it or eating too much increases stress on the stomach and is an extremely bad idea.

Chapter Two

What to Eat

Now that you know the four stages of recovery and the basic diet to follow after undergoing a gastric bypass, let's focus on nutrition. A common aspect of this diet's stages is that they prescribe only wholesome and nutritious ingredients. Remember, your body has undergone quite a change, and it will severely restrict how much or what you can eat and drink. Do not get discouraged; instead, focus on all the foods you can eat to make yourself feel better. Here are some general dietary suggestions.

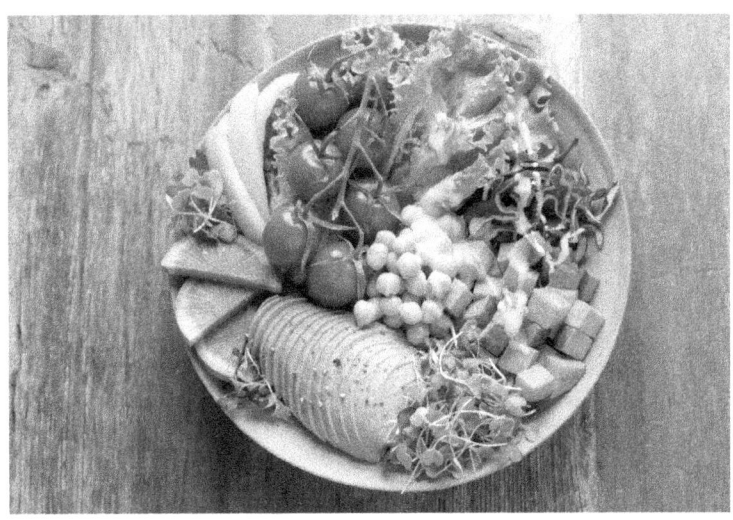

Dietary Suggestions for Stage 1

You must strictly follow a liquid diet during the first days. Apart from fluids, do not consume anything else. Broth, 1% or skimmed milk, decaffeinated coffee or tea, and unsweetened juices are ideal during the first stage of recovery. You are required to drink only clear liquids during the first and second days after surgery, and broth is the best choice.

Dietary Suggestions for Stage 2

Once you have made it through stage one, your body can fully tolerate liquids. During the second stage, you can start adding pureed and strained foods to your diet. Ensure that there are no solid pieces in it; the food's consistency must be similar to that of a smooth paste or thick liquid. The most common items that can be reintroduced in this stage include lean ground meat, fish, cooked cereal, soft cheese, sauces and gravies, cooked fruits and vegetables without skin, creamy soups, and soft scrambled eggs. You can still drink other liquids such as broth, sugar-free juices, and skimmed milk. Avoid pre-packaged juices.

Dietary Suggestions for Stage 3

Now that you have made it to the third stage, you can start reintroducing soft foods. Before doing this, don't forget to consult your healthcare provider. The foods you opt for must be easy to chew and soft. You can opt for ground meat, poultry without skin, cooked cereal, dry cereal with milk, soft fruit without skin and seeds, fully cooked vegetables without skin, and some rice. If you notice any discomfort after eating certain foods, avoid them for the time being.

Dietary Suggestions for Stage 4

By now, your body is fully capable of digesting the foods you were introduced to until now. During the fourth stage, you can reintroduce firm or solid foods. However, you need to do it slowly. You can consume at least three meals consisting of a solid food body. Each meal you eat should not be more than a quarter to one cup of cooked food. Don't reintroduce different ingredients at once. Instead, give a gap of at least 3-5 days before introducing a new ingredient. This gives you a chance to see whether your body can fully adjust to what you are eating or not. Avoid raw vegetables, any fibrous vegetables even if they're cooked, fried foods, tough meats including fatty cuts, highly seasoned or spicy foods, all types of bread, carbonated and caffeinated beverages, nuts and seeds, and popcorn. If you have any doubt about whether you can or cannot eat a single ingredient, ensure that you consult your healthcare provider immediately.

Apart from all the dietary suggestions mentioned until now, you need to drink around 2 liters or 64 ounces of fluids per day to prevent dehydration.

What to Avoid

In the previous section, you were introduced to different foods that you can safely consume after a gastric bypass. In this section, let's look at the different foods you must avoid.

Stay away from foods that are filled with empty calories. You must understand that the size of your stomach shrinks after the surgery, and you cannot eat as you did before. This is because the nutrients your body requires will be obtained from the food you eat. So, unless you make healthy and wise dietary choices, the chance of obtaining the needed nutrients reduces. Some common foods that are rich in calories but devoid of nutrients include fried foods, pastries, cakes and biscuits, and all other sorts of junk foods, along with sugar-laden treats. If your usual diet is rich in all these items, your calorie intake increases without the needed nutrients. This is the quickest way to put on weight. This also increases the risk of dumping syndrome. Dumping syndrome occurs when you quickly eat or eat more than you should after undergoing a gastric bypass.

Dietary fiber is often recommended for better digestion. After undergoing bypass surgery, foods rich in dietary fiber must be avoided. Fiber is not only difficult to digest but increases the stress on the newly stapled stomach too. So, some common foods you must avoid include cruciferous vegetables, corn, and fiber-rich fruits. This is also one of the reasons why the skin or peel and seeds of fruits and vegetables must be removed before consumption. Once your body is getting used to solid foods, you can slowly try reintroducing these ingredients and train your body to tolerate them. However, for now, it is better to avoid all such foods.

If you carefully go through the four stages of the gastric bypass diet and the foods allowed, one thing becomes abundantly clear: dry foods are introduced only at the end. During the initial stage of the diet, avoid all dry foods. This is because you are not allowed to drink water while eating, and swallowing dry food can become difficult. Even if you want to opt for dry foods such as cereals or granola, ensure that they are softened with low-fat milk or a dairy alternative of your choosing.

Avoid alcohol after undergoing a gastric bypass. Alcohol is not only rich in empty calories, but also your body's ability to absorb alcohol increases significantly after the surgery. Similarly, stay away from all carbonated and caffeinated beverages. Such beverages are usually associated with an increased risk of dumping syndrome. Caffeine also increases the risk of dehydration. So, avoiding the above-mentioned drinks is better for your overall health and recovery. It is also better to opt for calorie-free and unsweetened beverages.

During postoperative recovery, stay away from fatty and tough cuts of meat. Slowly and thoroughly chewing the food before swallowing is an essential and helpful eating habit to develop. This is doubly important if you have undergone bariatric surgery. The more thoroughly you chew before swallowing, the easier it is for your body to digest it. Tough meats are usually difficult to chew and are therefore best avoided. The foods you eat shouldn't have any gristle or fat, especially during the initial stages when you are slowly readjusting to chewing.

You must be mindful of the fats consumed after undergoing a gastric bypass. Fatty and deep-fried foods are filled with unhealthy calories. Consuming them can increase the occurrence of certain unpleasant symptoms such as nausea and vomiting. Understand that your stomach and the intestinal tract are quite sensitive right now. Consuming any foods that can cause inflammation or irritation isn't a good decision. Similarly, steer clear of all deli and processed meats. Whether it is burgers, bacon, sausages, or salami, stay away from them. Try to consume fresh ingredients and home-cooked meals as much as possible. A little extra effort, especially toward the diet you follow, will significantly improve your health.

After going through the list of food items you must avoid, one thing becomes clear: all unhealthy foods are automatically eliminated from your diet. This is one of the best ways to ensure that you eat healthily, not just for now but throughout your life.

Chapter Three

Tips to Remember

Until now, you were introduced to different nutritional requirements while following the gastric bypass diet after surgery. During this point, the primary focus is not just on recovery but also on developing healthy and lifelong eating habits as well. It's the only way to reap the benefits of the surgery and maintain them. This section will introduce you to tips and suggestions you must always remember while eating.

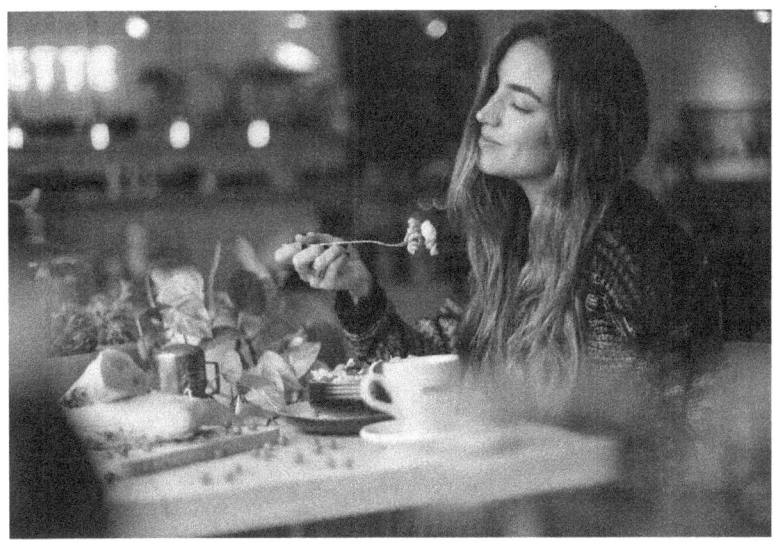

Do you usually grab a bite before heading to work in the morning? Or do you eat quickly? If yes, you need to change this habit. Eating quickly is extremely harmful and will get in the way of recovery after undergoing a gastric bypass. Instead, give yourself anywhere between 20-30 minutes per meal. Sit comfortably and eat slowly. It doesn't matter, even if it is an extremely small meal. You will need time because you will have to chew every bite thoroughly. The simplest way to ensure that you are eating slowly is by taking small bites. Initially, it's better to start with bites the size of a pencil eraser. Slowly, you can move on to slightly bigger bites. Don't forget to chew thoroughly before swallowing. Do not gulp, and do not take big bites. If there's something you cannot chew properly, then do not swallow it. This is one of the reasons why fatty and tough meats must be avoided.

A simple habit you must learn is avoiding eating and drinking simultaneously. As a rule of thumb, avoid drinking anything 30 minutes before and after eating. This will give your newly stapled stomach the time needed to process the food consumed without any unnecessary stress on it.

Mindfulness is a brilliant practice that will come in handy in all aspects of life, not just your diet. Mindfulness essentially refers to the ability to stay fully engaged and focused on the present. It is about staying focused only on the task at hand and nothing else. Are you used to eating while watching television or something else? Do you end up overeating because of this? Well, now is the time to change all this. This is where mindfulness steps into the picture. When you are eating mindfully, you will be fully focused only on the food on your plate and nothing else. This will make it easier to understand your body's cues of satiety and fullness. If you end up eating too much or too quickly, it can disrupt the staples in the stomach, cause nausea and vomiting, or trigger terrible pain under the breastbone.

Other than the four-stage approach you were introduced to for slowly reintroducing foods, be mindful of the portion sizes too. This will be one of the significant changes you need to make. You can no longer eat like you used to. Gastric bypass surgery shrinks the size of the stomach. As you recover from it, the stomach also stretches a little but not much. So, it can only hold a little food at any given point. Therefore, measuring the portions you eat is a wonderful idea. Measure the portions and don't overeat. This is a great way to ensure that your daily nutritional quota is met. Small meals are your friend during recovery. Aim to eat around 4-6 meals per day instead of three big meals. For the initial two months following the surgery, please stick to the gastric bypass diet without any deviations. Small plates and bowls make it easier to stick to the portion sizes. During the first two months after the surgery, your daily calorie intake must be between 300 and 600 calories and no more. All of it must be derived from thin and thick liquids.

To avoid dehydration, you need to drink at least two liters or eight cups of water daily. However, avoid drinking too much around mealtime because it will leave you feeling full and prevent the consumption of the needed nutrients. Ideally, sip on a cup of liquid of your choice in between the meals consumed to avoid dehydration. Ensure that you do this 6-8 times daily to maintain the needed hydration.

Avoid using straws for drinking. This can introduce air into the newly stapled stomach pouch and cause physical discomfort.

Once you have a dietary plan on hand, ensure that you stick to it. Also, ensure that you consult your healthcare provider before making any dietary changes. Take some time and go through all the different recipes given in this book. You can easily make a nutritious and wholesome meal plan using these recipes.

Since the portions of the food you consume will reduce, focusing on nutrient-dense foods is a must. You will need to add some supplements to prevent nutritional deficiencies. Consult your healthcare provider and add them. Accordingly, the most common multivitamins you will be prescribed will include iron, folic acid, copper, zinc, selenium, and copper. You might also need vitamin D, calcium, and vitamin B12 supplements.

After a while, you can slowly increase the variety and consistency of the foods consumed. That said, you might not be able to tolerate some foods you could before the surgery. However, this isn't something to worry about. Some common foods that belong to this category include fruits and vegetables rich in fiber, bread, and red meat. Usually, the daily calorie intake prescribed in the long run is around 1000 per day. You will need to consume well-balanced meals that include all food groups. Apart from this, you must still drink at least two liters of water to stay hydrated.

Chapter Four

The Road to Recovery and Better Health

Undergoing the operation and transitioning to solid foods is a significant victory! You are a post-op bariatric warrior! Congratulations on making it to this stage. Now, the primary focus must be on regaining your good health, optimizing it, and leaving unhealthy food habits in the past. Whether you live by yourself or have a family, you will need to make a couple of healthy changes from now on. The good news is that these changes are not only practical but easy to make as well. Once you get into the habit of prioritizing your health, you will not want to go back to unhealthy eating habits.

Tips to a Speedy Recovery

Focusing on your body's recovery is crucial. That said, your body underwent a significant change, which isn't without any side effects. The most common complications you must prepare yourself for include dehydration and malnutrition. Apart from this, another common side effect is known as the dumping syndrome. Follow the simple suggestions given in this section to deal with the above-mentioned side effects of the surgery successfully.

Maintain a Food Journal

The first thing you must do is keep track of everything you eat and drink daily. This is one of the healthiest food habits you can develop, and there is no time like the present to do it. The idea of journaling or recording everything you eat and drink is to become conscious of what and how much you eat. It's not about restricting yourself. Instead, it's about becoming mindful. Remember, your stomach is still healing and recovering, and you should not stress it any further. Weighing the food and tracking the portion size is the best way to ensure that you are not increasing the stress on the recovering stomach.

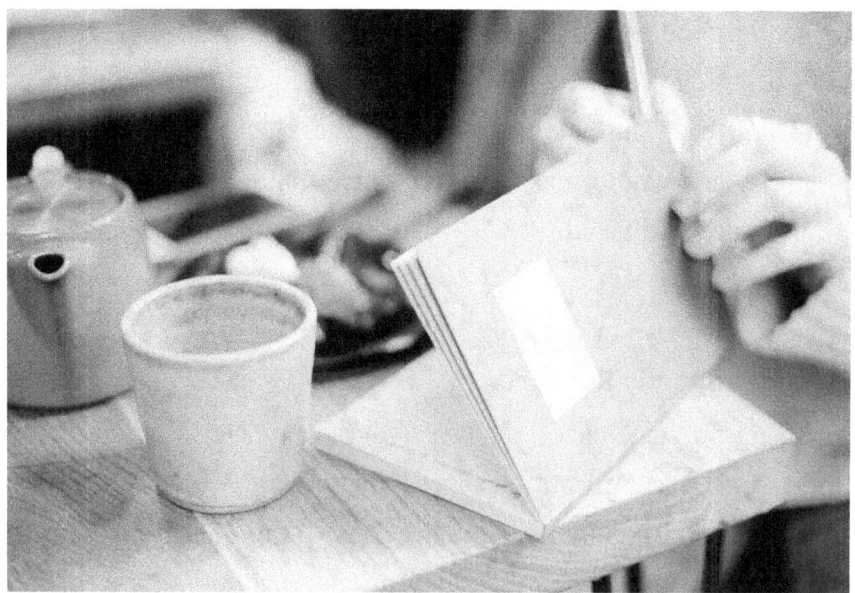

Tackle Dehydration

As mentioned, one of the most common symptoms of undergoing gastric bypass surgery is dehydration. If you do not drink sufficient fluids, it results in a condition known as dehydration. It's commonly characterized by thirstiness and reduction in the frequency of urination or the urine taking on a dark yellow color. Even though the new stomach can hold only a small amount of fluid at once, it doesn't mean you do not drink sufficient water. As a rule of thumb, you need up to 64 ounces or two liters of fluids per day. This is equal to approximately 8 cups of water. Ensure that the fluids you opt for are not carbonated and free of sugar and caffeine. While drinking, do not gulp it down; instead, drink slowly. Avoid using straws or drinking out of the bottles because it can cause painful digestive gas. Along the same lines, avoid carbonated beverages for the first couple of months. Another tip you must remember while drinking any fluid is to separate it from your mealtimes. Drinking anything while eating increases the risk of improper digestion.

Be Mindful of Protein Consumption

Protein is one of the most important micronutrients for your overall health. It is considered to be the building block of muscles. Also, it is an extremely crucial part of the new diet you will be following after the surgery. Protein is needed to increase satiety levels and ensure your body's regular working. In fact, after surgery, most surgical teams recommend the consumption of protein shakes daily. As a rule of thumb, the meals you consume must be low and fat and rich in protein-filled foods. You need to consume between 60 and 100 grams of protein per day. If you usually eat meat, avoid meats that are tough or full of unhealthy fats. Instead, it's better to opt for chopped meat. As mentioned, do not swallow any food you cannot chew thoroughly. Doing this simply results in a blocked stoma. Avoid proteins rich in fat, such as processed and pre-packaged deli meats, including sausages, cold cuts, bacon, and so on. Instead, opt for food sources rich in protein and low in fats, such as chicken and turkey, fish and shellfish, eggs, fat-free or low-fat dairy products, tofu and soy milk, and peanut butter. Even though plant-based foods such as beans, lentils, and veggies contain protein, they contain high levels of dietary fiber that your body doesn't need right now. If you cannot meet the daily protein requirement or are struggling to do so, consult your healthcare provider and add a protein supplement to the daily diet. If you are lactose intolerant, be careful about the dietary supplement you are adding. Not consuming enough protein includes tiredness, excess hair loss, and dry skin. Even though some of these symptoms are common after undergoing a gastric bypass, optimizing the protein intake helps reduce their intensity.

One Ingredient at a Time

After surgery, certain foods can cause nausea, blockage, abdominal pain, discomfort, and vomiting too. The most common foods that cause the symptoms mentioned above include fruits and vegetables, carbs such as bread and pasta, and fatty meats. If you wish to add any of these ingredients to your diet, do it slowly, one ingredient at a time. If you cannot tolerate any of them, try reintroducing them 1-2 weeks later. Also, dairy products are one of the most common ingredients you need to be extra careful about while reintroducing.

Any problem digesting or tolerating lactose can increase after surgery, so opting for lactose-free products is a good idea.

Deal with Dumping Syndrome

A condition that usually occurs after undergoing gastric bypass surgery is the dumping syndrome. It essentially refers to the rapid entry of sugar-rich meals into the intestine directly from the stomach pouch. This is where it gets the name "dumping" from. This usually happens within 10-30 minutes of consuming sugar-rich foods. At times, it can take up to 2-3 hours after eating as well. The dumping syndrome occurs if you eat too much at once or are eating too quickly. The most common symptoms associated with it include elevated heart rate, cramping in the intestinal and abdominal area, nausea and vomiting, dizziness, sweating, and diarrhea. Usually, the symptoms can pass between 15-30 minutes of occurring. Most of these symptoms disappear if you slowly sip a cup of water. In some instances, the symptoms can go on for a few hours and make you feel anxious and shaky.

The most common cause of this syndrome is food rich in sugar. Sticking to a low-sugar diet is a great way to improve your overall health. It means you must avoid foods rich in sugars, such as sweetened yogurt, juices, cereals, ice creams, chocolates, candies, dried and preserved fruit, and anything that has sugar added to it. Apart from this, avoid sugary beverages such as fruit juices, sodas, coffee, or tea flavored with sugar, all artificial sweeteners, and all sugary condiments. As a rule of thumb, make it a point to carefully read through the list of ingredients before purchasing any food items. Anything that contains sugar, artificial sweeteners, or even natural sweeteners such as honey must be avoided.

Vitamin and Mineral Supplements

After undergoing any bariatric surgery, the different nutrients your body requires cannot be efficiently absorbed from the food consumed. The most common problems caused by a low intake of vitamins and minerals include sores around the mouth, tiredness, and anemia. Over a period, if your body doesn't get the required vitamins and minerals it needs, it results in other health conditions and complications. Depending on the recommendation of your healthcare provider, a vitamin or mineral supplement must be added to your daily routine.

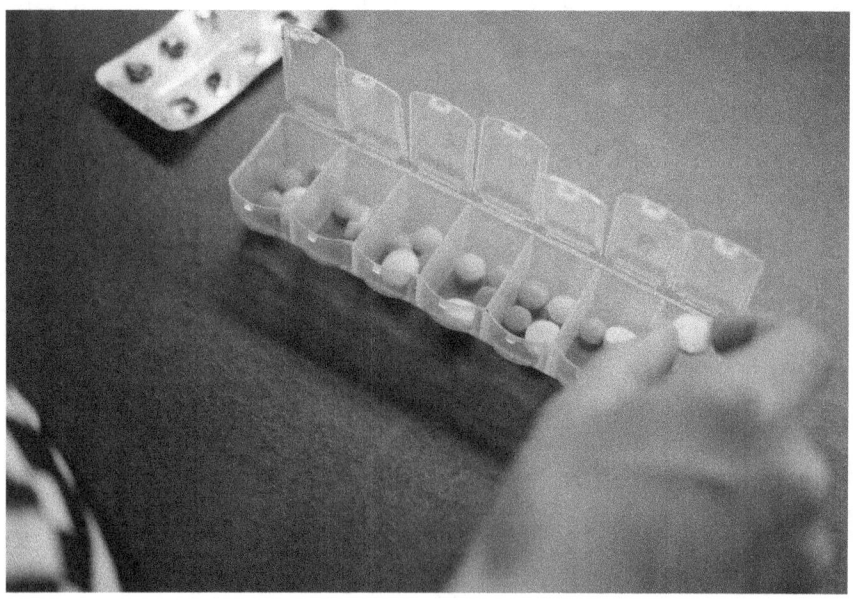

Keep an Open Mind

Apart from all this, ensure that you keep an open mind about this diet. Instead of fixating on all things you cannot eat, concentrate on the ones you can. Also, you just need to make it through the first couple of weeks. After this, you can slowly start reintroducing the solid foods you used to eat. With a little planning and preparation, sticking to this diet becomes easy. Your attitude toward the diet you follow matters because it determines your motivation to stick to it. Focusing on all you can eat reduces the chances of developing a limiting mindset. Also, with a little creativity, you can easily recreate healthier versions of all the foods you loved and enjoyed before undergoing surgery.

Tips for Successful Meal Planning

This book introduces you to different recipes that can be used while recovering from the gastric bypass. Organization and planning are the two essential tools needed for post-op weight loss and recovery. Without these things, recovery becomes difficult. Remember, it is not about sacrificing flavor and taste for the sake of health. Instead, it is about a little planning that ensures you are eating different meals daily and are not getting bored. This is where the concept of meal planning steps into the picture. It refers to deciding on the meals you wish to cook based on the available ingredients and your preferences. Once you know what you want to eat, gathering the required ingredients becomes easy. Meal planning is a great way to cut down on your food budget, cook healthy and wholesome meals, avoid repetition, and stick to a dietary regimen.

Here are some tips for meal planning.

Portioning the Meals

The portion size is the most important aspect of the diet you need to focus on after gastric bypass. You will be consuming small portions instead of regular-sized ones. If you are used to eating three big meals daily, you'll need to condition your body slowly to eat six smaller meals instead. While planning, you can cook regular-sized portions and then divide them into smaller ones ideal for your diet. Once the portions are in place, simply store them in individual containers or packets. After this, consume whatever you want to and freeze the rest. You can cook a recipe you like at once and store it for later. This makes cooking over the weekdays quite simple. The meals simply need to be removed from the freezer, heated, and then served.

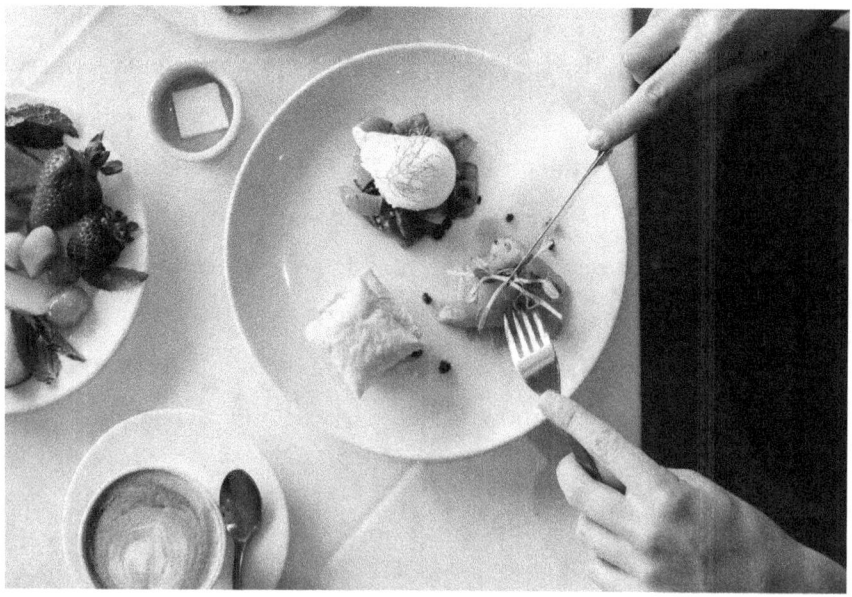

Keep It Interesting

An extremely important aspect of meal planning is ensuring your meals don't become boring and repetitive. The willingness to stick to a diet will obviously reduce if you need to eat the same food day in and out. So, once you have made up your mind about this diet, pick a selection of recipes. Try to include as much variety as possible. You can also cycle the menu after a couple of weeks. Knowing that you will be eating foods that appeal to you makes it easier to stick to a diet. The good news is that you don't have to spend time searching for recipes to fit your dietary requirements. Instead, simply go through the ones given in this book.

While planning, take stock of all the ingredients you have at home and the ones to be purchased. This is a great way to keep track of your grocery bills too. As much as possible, try to opt for seasonal ingredients. They are not only cheaper but are more flavorful too.

Make the Most of the Weekends

Whenever you have some time available or over the weekend, spend a couple of hours planning and prepping meals. This involves batch cooking proteins, cutting vegetables and fruits, or even cooking sauces, stews, soups, and curries. Before doing this, you need to spend some time and make a list of meals you wish to consume over the following week or a couple of days. Once the recipes are in place, make a note of all the ingredients needed. Simply prep whatever you can and store. For instance, if most of the recipes you have opted for include lean protein such as skinless chicken or turkey, tofu, or fish, you can prepare them in a large batch. Once the protein is cooked, simply add the other fixings and you have a good meal.

While prepping, consider the cooking time involved too. Start with items with the longest cooking time. Whether it is roasting vegetables, cooking protein, or making a stew, they are time-consuming steps. Once you get such elements out of the way, cooking becomes quite easy during the week.

It Is Okay to Eat Out

One thing you must understand is that it is perfectly okay to eat out. That said, you need to be extra careful whenever you eat out. The one thing you must not forget is to stay away from the list of ingredients discussed in the previous chapter. For instance, avoiding red meats and deep-fried foods after undergoing gastric bypass is recommended. Therefore, French fries or a burger from the drive-thru are automatically eliminated. Instead, you can opt for a simple protein salad. Whenever you have to eat out, carefully go through all the different items on the menu and select something that fits the gastric bypass diet. More importantly, pay attention to the ingredients you should not be eating and stay away from them.

Quick and Smart Cooking Options

There will be days when you neither have the time nor the energy to prepare elaborate meals. Or days when you are hungry but don't want to rely on takeout. You can prepare healthy and delicious meals even on such days with little planning. Here are three little suggestions that will make things easy.

The first thing you must do is always keep a few portions of frozen vegetables in the freezer. Apart from this, you will also need a couple of easy-to-cook proteins on your hands, such as skinless chicken breast, tuna, or tofu. Heat the frozen veggies and serve it with a side of lean protein of your choice and a low-cal dressing for some flavor. And voila, a healthy and tasty meal is ready within a couple of minutes. All this is possible only with a little planning and preparation.

Have a couple of nutrient-dense ready-to-eat food options such as low-fat cheese and Greek yogurt. A small bowl of natural Greek yogurt coupled with a sprinkling of whole-grain cereal or a portion of low-fat cheese served with some fruit without skin makes for excellent small meals. These are not only easy to prepare but are tasty and give your body the needed energy.

Finally, take some time over the weekends, as mentioned above, to batch cook certain foods. Whether it is a soup, stew, or curry of your choice, go ahead and do it. So, on busy days, you simply need to thaw it, and the meal is ready within no time! Another important aspect of meal planning and prepping is investing in the right storage containers. Food will stay fresh only when it is stored properly. You can use Ziplock bags, freezer-friendly containers and bags, and other similar storage containers.

Apart from all the suggestions mentioned above, don't hesitate to consult your healthcare provider or dietician for further help. They will give you the information needed to help devise a meal plan that caters to your needs and requirements. Also, if you have any doubts, don't hesitate to reach out to your healthcare provider.

NOTE: Before you decide to incorporate any of the suggestions discussed in all the chapters mentioned until now, consult your healthcare provider. Ensure that the meals you wish to consume will promote recovery and healing instead of hindering it. Also, if you notice any reactions after consuming certain food, consult medical help immediately.

Chapter Five

Gastric Bypass Smoothie Recipes

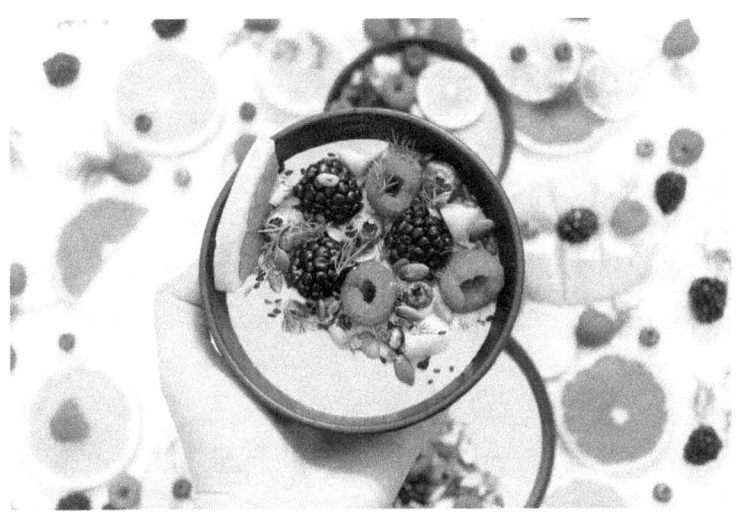

Note:

- Always wash the fruits and vegetables well before chopping.
- It is advisable to have the smoothie within an hour of preparing it. Once you prepare the smoothie, let it rest for 5 to 10 minutes before consuming it. The air bubbles will deflate, helping prevent bloating.

- If you find the smoothie very thick, feel free to add more liquid or water and dilute it. You can also pour thick smoothies into a bowl and eat them as a smoothie bowl.

- Adding a scoop or two of protein powder to the smoothie will help you recover faster.

- You can add ice cubes while blending.

Stage /Phase 2: Liquid and pureed diet (Generally 15 – 30 days after surgery but it can vary)

Banana Cream Protein Shake

Serves: 1

Ingredients:

- 1 ¼ scoops vanilla whey protein powder
- 1/3 teaspoon vanilla extract
- 2/3 teaspoon banana extract
- 1 ¼ cups water or unsweetened almond milk

Directions:

1. Pour water or milk into the blender.
2. Add protein powder, vanilla extract, and banana extract and blend until well combined.
3. Pour into a glass and serve with crushed ice.

Stage /Phase 3: Soft diet (Generally between 5 – 12 weeks after surgery but it can vary)

Avocado Smoothie

Serves: 1

Ingredients:

- 1 ripe banana
- ¼ avocado, peeled, mashed
- Ice cubes, as required
- ½ teaspoon vanilla extract
- 1 cup coconut water
- 1 tablespoon honey or stevia drops to taste (optional)
- ½ teaspoon ground cinnamon
- A pinch of salt

Directions:

1. Add banana, avocado, cinnamon, and water into a blender.
2. Blend the mixture until you get a smooth puree.
3. Add ice cubes, vanilla extract, honey, and salt and blend once again for a few seconds until well incorporated.
4. Pour into a tall glass and serve.

Berry Oatmeal Smoothie

Serves: 1

Ingredients:

- 2 teaspoons oatmeal
- 1/8 cup raspberries
- 1/8 cup blueberries
- ¼ cup nonfat milk
- 2 inches ripe banana, chopped
- Sweetener like stevia or swerve to taste (optional)

Directions:

1. Cook the raspberries and blueberries in a small saucepan until they burst. Turn off the heat and let it cool completely.
2. Place the oatmeal, raspberry/blueberry mixture, banana, and oatmeal in a blender.
3. Pour milk over the ingredients in the blender.
4. Blend the mixture until you get a smooth puree.
5. Pour into a glass and serve.

Gingerbread Smoothie

Serves: 2

Ingredients:

- 2 cups nonfat milk or unsweetened almond milk
- ½ teaspoon ground nutmeg
- 2 teaspoons ground ginger
- 2 bananas, sliced, frozen
- 2 tablespoons plain nonfat Greek yogurt
- 4 scoops protein powder
- Ice cubes, as required

Directions:

1. Add nutmeg, ginger, bananas, yogurt, protein powder, and ice cubes into a blender. Pour milk and blend until smooth.

2. Pour into glasses and serve. You can consume one glass of the smoothie and freeze the remaining in ice cube trays or Popsicle molds.

3. Towards the end of this stage, if your doctor permits, you can add almond butter or peanut butter while making the smoothie.

Stage /Phase 4: Regular diet (Generally after 12 weeks after surgery but it can vary)

Powerhouse Smoothie

Serves: 1 large glass or 2 smaller glasses

Ingredients:

- 1/8 cup hemp seeds
- ½ ripe banana, sliced
- ¼ cup pomegranate arils, fresh or frozen
- 2 cups fresh salad greens or spinach or collard greens or lightly steamed kale
- 1 tablespoon cocoa powder, unsweetened
- ½ tablespoon ground chia seeds
- Juice of ½ lime
- 1 ½ cups filtered water
- ½ cup frozen strawberries
- ½ inch fresh ginger, peeled, sliced
- A handful fresh mint leaves
- 1 tablespoon flax meal
- ¼ cup frozen raw broccoli florets

Directions:

1. Add hemp seeds and about ½ cup of water into the blender.

2. Blend on high speed for about 15 seconds.

3. Add banana, pomegranate, and strawberries and blend for a few more seconds.

4. Add salad greens, cocoa, chia seeds, lime juice, ginger, mint leaves, flax meal, and broccoli into the blender. Pour remaining water.

5. You can steam the broccoli florets if desired.

6. Blend for 30 -40 seconds or until smooth.

7. Pour into a tall glass and serve.

8. Serve right away.

Watermelon Strawberry Smoothie

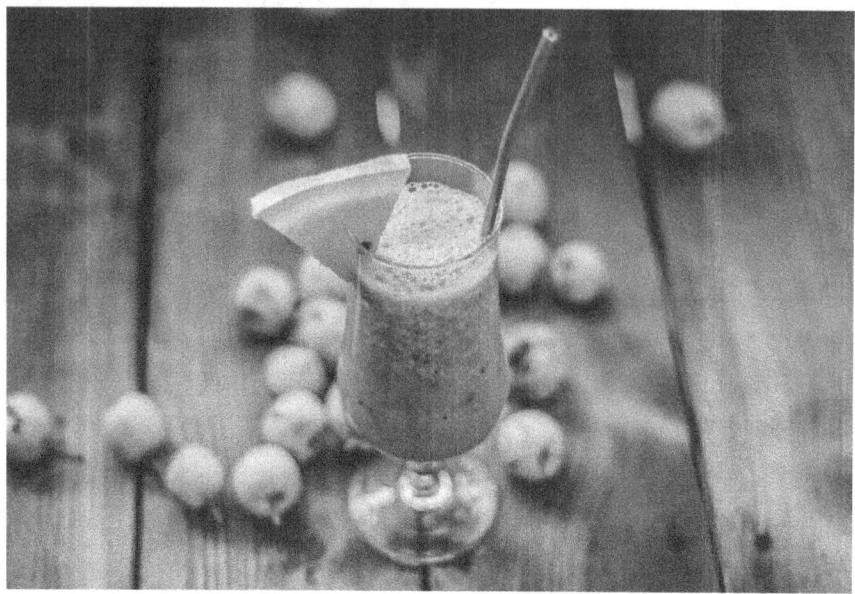

Serves: 2

Ingredients:

- 1 cup nonfat milk or almond milk, soy milk or rice milk
- 2 packets Bari Life's Vanilla protein pudding/shake or strawberry protein pudding shake mix (optional)
- 6 strawberries, fresh or frozen
- Ice cubes, as required
- 2 cups cubed, deseeded watermelon
- 4 – 5 mint leaves (optional)
- 2 scoops Bari Life Complete Bariatric Vitamin Powder – Watermelon

Directions:

1. Add vanilla protein pudding, strawberries, ice, watermelon, mint leaves, and Bariatric vitamin powder into a blender. Pour milk over the ingredients and blend until smooth.

2. Pour into glasses and serve. You can consume one glass of the smoothie and freeze the remaining in ice cube trays or Popsicle molds.

Superfood Rainbow Smoothie

Serves: 1

Ingredients:

For blue/purple layer:

- 1/3 cup frozen blueberries
- 1/8 cup nonfat milk or almond milk
- ½ tablespoon peanut butter or almond butter

For green layer:

- ¼ ripe avocado, peeled, pitted, chopped
- ½ cup fresh baby spinach
- ½ banana, sliced, frozen

For dark pink/purple layer:

- ½ cup frozen strawberries
- ½ cup frozen pitted cherries
- 1/8 cup nonfat milk or almond milk
- ¼ teaspoon vanilla extract

For yellow layer:

- 2/3 cup frozen mango
- 2 inches banana
- 2 tablespoons nonfat milk or almond milk

For pink layer:

- ½ cup frozen raspberries
- 1/8 cup nonfat milk or almond milk
- 1 tablespoon hemp hearts

Optional toppings: Use any

- Kiwi slices
- Blueberries
- Cherries
- Strawberry slices
- Peach slices
- Light whipped topping
- Sprinkles etc.

Directions:

1. For the blue layer, blend blueberries, milk, and almond butter in a blender until smooth and thick.

2. Pour the smoothie into a glass. Place the glass in the freezer. Clean the blender.

3. For the dark pink/purple layer: Blend together strawberries, cherries, vanilla, and milk in a blender until smooth and thick. Pour it gently over the blue layer.

4. Place the glass in the freezer. Clean the blender.

5. For the green layer, blend avocado, spinach, and banana in a blender until smooth and thick. Pour it gently over the dark pink/purple layer.

6. Place the glass in the freezer. Clean the blender.

7. For the yellow layer, blend mango, banana, and milk together in a blender until smooth and thick. Pour the smoothie gently over the green layer. Place the glass in the freezer. Clean the blender.

8. For the pink layer, blend raspberries, milk, and hemp hearts in a blender. Blend for 30-40 seconds or until smooth and thick.

9. Pour the smoothie gently over the yellow layer. Place the glass in the freezer for 15-20 minutes.

10. Top with the optional serving options and serve.

Orange Lemonade Smoothie

Serves: 2

Ingredients:

- 3 ounces fresh orange juice
- 2 bananas, sliced, frozen
- 2 scoops Bari Life Complete Bariatric Vitamin Powder – Lemonade
- 2 packets Bari's Life's Aloha mango protein smoothie mix
- 2 – 3 cups spinach
- Juice of 2 lemons
- Ice cubes as required
- Water as required

Directions:

1. Blend orange juice, bananas, Bariatric vitamin powder, mango protein smoothie mix, spinach, lemon juice, ice cubes, and water in a blender until smooth.

2. Pour into 2 glasses and serve. You can consume one glass of the smoothie and freeze the remaining in ice cube trays or Popsicle molds.

Green Cleansing Smoothie

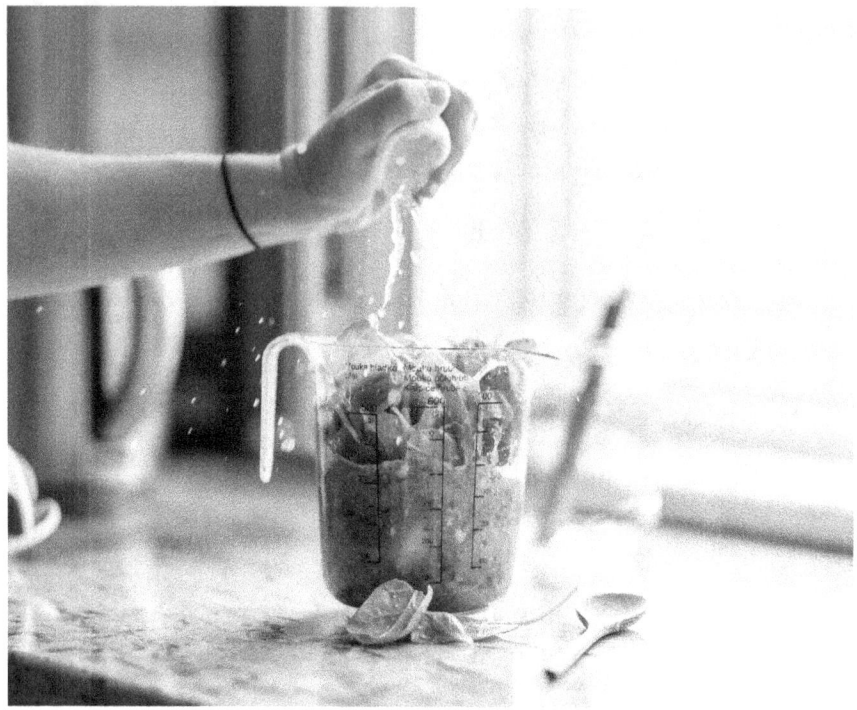

Serves: 2

Ingredients:

- 2 cups spinach or kale leaves, torn, discard hard stems and ribs
- 1 cup chopped cucumber
- 1 large pear, cored, chopped
- A handful mint leaves
- 2 tablespoons lemon juice or to taste
- ½ inch piece fresh ginger, peeled, sliced

- ¼ teaspoon ground cinnamon (optional)
- ¼ teaspoon turmeric powder (optional)
- A pinch cayenne pepper (optional)
- 2 bananas, sliced, frozen
- 1 cup chopped celery
- 2 cups romaine lettuce
- A handful fresh parsley
- 1 teaspoon chia seeds
- 2 cups coconut water or water
- Natural sweetener like stevia or honey (optional) to taste

Directions:

1. Blend spinach, kale, bananas, celery, pears, lettuce, parsley, mint, cucumber, lemon juice, chia seeds, turmeric powder, coconut water, sweetener, cinnamon, and cayenne pepper in a blender until smooth.

2. Blend for 30-40 seconds or until smooth.

3. Add more coconut water if you like a smoothie of a thinner consistency.

4. Pour into tall glasses and serve with crushed ice.

Blueberry Lemonade Smoothie

Serves: 2

Ingredients:

- 6 ounces fresh or frozen blueberries
- Juice of 2 lemons
- 2 scoops Bari Life Complete Bariatric Vitamin Powder – Lemonade
- 2 – 3 cups spinach
- 1 banana, sliced, frozen
- 2 packets Bari's Life's Berry delicious protein smoothie mix or vanilla protein pudding/shake mix
- Ice cubes as required
- 2 teaspoons chia seeds
- Stevia drops to taste (optional)
- 2 cups water or more if required

Directions:

1. Blend blueberries, banana, Bariatric vitamin powder, protein smoothie mix, spinach, lemon juice, ice cubes, chia seeds, stevia, and water in a blender until smooth.

2. Pour into 2 glasses and serve. You can consume one glass of the smoothie and freeze the remaining in ice cube trays or Popsicle molds.

Carrot Smoothie

Serves: 2

Ingredients:

- 8 carrots, peeled, chopped
- Juice of 2 lemons
- 2 scoops Bari Life Complete Bariatric Vitamin Powder – Lemonade
- ½ bunch parsley
- 2 bananas, sliced, frozen
- 1-inch piece of ginger, peeled, sliced
- Ice cubes as required
- 6 teaspoons hemp seeds
- Stevia drops to taste (optional)
- 2 cups water or more if required

Directions:

1. Blend carrots, banana, Bariatric vitamin powder, parsley, lemon juice, ice cubes, hemp seeds, stevia, and water in a blender until smooth.

2. Pour into 2 glasses and serve. You can consume one glass of the smoothie and freeze the remaining in ice cube trays or Popsicle molds.

Berry, Banana and Kale Smoothie

Serves: 1

Ingredients:

For banana and almond layer:

- 1 small banana, peeled, sliced
- ½ cup nonfat milk
- ¼ cup crushed ice
- 5 almonds

For kale and date layer:

- 1 Medjool date, pitted, chopped
- 1/8 cup crushed ice
- 1 cup chopped kale, discard hard stem and ribs, torn

For blueberry layer:

- A handful blueberries
- ¼ cup crushed ice
- 1/8 cup water
- 1 teaspoon flaxseed meal or protein powder

For strawberry layer:

- 3 – 4 strawberries, hulled
- ½ cup crushed ice

- 1/8 cup nonfat milk

- 1 teaspoon flaxseed meal or protein powder

Directions:

1. For the banana and almond layer: Blend banana, almond, milk, and ice into a blender. Blend for 30-40 seconds or until smooth and thick.

2. Pour the smoothie into a glass. Place the glass in the freezer. Clean the blender.

3. For the kale and date layer: Add kale, dates, and ice into a blender. Blend for 30-40 seconds or until smooth and thick.

4. Pour the smoothie gently over the banana and almond layer gently. Clean the blender.

5. For the blueberry layer: Add blueberries, ice, water, and flaxseed meal into a blender. Blend for 30-40 seconds or until smooth and thick.

6. Gently pour the smoothie over the kale and date layer. Place the glass in the freezer. Clean the blender.

7. For the strawberry layer: Add strawberries, ice, milk, and flaxseed meal into a blender. Blend for 30-40 seconds or until smooth and thick.

8. Pour the smoothie gently over the blueberry layer.

9. Serve right away.

Avocado and Papaya Smoothie

Serves: 2

Ingredients:

- 2 cups green tea, chilled
- 1 cup fresh or frozen papaya chunks
- 1 cup fresh or frozen blueberries
- 2/3 medium avocado, peeled, pitted, chopped
- 2 tablespoon chia seeds
- 1 teaspoon turmeric powder
- 1-inch piece ginger, peeled, sliced
- 2 scoops protein powder
- 1 teaspoon cinnamon powder
- 1/8 teaspoon salt
- ½ teaspoon cayenne pepper
- 2 teaspoons honey or maple syrup or stevia drops to taste
- 1 cup pitted fresh or frozen cherries, (optional)
- 2 cups baby spinach (optional)

Directions:

1. Add blueberries, papaya, avocado, chia seeds, turmeric powder, ginger, protein powder, cayenne pepper, green tea, cinnamon, salt, honey, cherries, and spinach if using it in a blender. Blend until smooth.

2. Pour into tall glasses and serve with crushed ice. You can consume one glass of the smoothie and freeze the remaining in ice cube trays or Popsicle molds.

Layered Banana Split Protein Smoothie

Serves: 1

Ingredients:

For the chocolate layer:

- ½ banana, sliced, frozen
- ¾ tablespoon unsweetened cocoa powder
- 1/8 cup nonfat milk or nondairy milk of your choice like almond milk, oat milk, soy milk, etc.
- 1 tablespoon vanilla protein powder
- ½ teaspoon chia seeds

For the banana layer:

- 1 tablespoon vanilla protein powder
- ½ banana, sliced, frozen
- 1/8 cup nonfat milk or nondairy milk of your choice like almond milk, oat milk, soy milk, etc.
- ½ teaspoon chia seeds

For the strawberry layer:

- 1 tablespoon vanilla protein powder
- 4 strawberries, frozen
- 1/8 cup nonfat milk or nondairy milk of your choice like almond milk, oat milk, soy milk, etc.

Directions:

1. To make the chocolate layer: Blend banana, cocoa, milk, protein powder, and chia seeds until smooth and thick.

2. Pour the smoothie into a glass. Place the glass in the freezer. Clean the blender.

3. To make the banana layer: Blend banana, milk, protein powder, and chia seeds until smooth and thick.

4. Pour the smoothie gently into the glass over the chocolate layer. Place the glass in the freezer. Clean the blender.

5. To make the strawberry layer: Add strawberries, milk, and protein powder into a blender and blend until smooth. Pour the smoothie over the banana layer. Place the glass in the freezer for 5 minutes.

6. Serve.

Orange Creamsicle Smoothie

Serves: 2

Ingredients:

- 2 oranges, peeled, separated into segments, deseeded
- Zest of 2 oranges, grated
- 1 cup plain nonfat Greek yogurt
- Ice cubes, as required
- 2 cups almond milk
- 2 scoops vanilla protein powder
- 2 teaspoons vanilla extract

Directions:

1. Add oranges, orange zest, yogurt, ice, milk, protein powder, and vanilla extract into a blender and blend until smooth.

2. Pour into glasses and serve. You can consume one glass of the smoothie and freeze the remaining in ice cube trays or Popsicle molds.

Pina Colada Protein Smoothie

Serves: 1

Ingredients:

- 1 ¼ cups unsweetened almond milk or nonfat milk
- 1/3 cup fresh or frozen pineapple pieces
- Ice cubes, as required
- 1 ½ tablespoons vanilla protein powder
- 3 tablespoons sugar-free coconut syrup

Directions:

1. Add milk, pineapple, ice cubes, protein powder, and coconut syrup into the blender and blend until smooth.
2. Pour into a glass and serve.

Raspberry Watermelon Mojito Smoothie

Serves: 2

Ingredients:

- 2 scoops vanilla protein powder
- 1 cup watermelon chunks
- Ice cubes, as required
- 2 cups water
- ¼ cup mint leaves
- ½ cup raspberries

Directions:

1. Add protein powder, watermelon, ice cubes, water, mint, and raspberries into a blender and blend until smooth.

2. Pour into glasses and serve. You can consume one glass of the smoothie and freeze the remaining in ice cube trays or Popsicle molds.

Layered Smoothie Bowl

Serves: 1

Ingredients:

For the mango layer:

- ½ cup frozen mango
- 1/3 cup coconut water or nonfat milk or almond milk
- 3 inches banana, sliced, frozen
- ½ scoop protein powder

For the berry layer:

- A handful fresh baby spinach (optional)
- 2/3 cup frozen mixed berries of your choice
- 1/3 cup coconut water or nonfat milk or almond milk
- ½ scoop protein powder

To serve:

- Banana slices
- Flaxseed meal
- Fresh fruit of your choice

Directions:

1. To make the mango layer: Blend mango, banana, protein powder, and milk in a blender until smooth.

2. Transfer the blended mixture into a bowl. Place the bowl in the freezer. Clean the blender.

3. To make the berry layer: Blend baby spinach, berries, coconut water, and protein powder in a blender until smooth.

4. Pour the smoothie carefully over the mango layer.

5. Top with banana slices and fresh fruits. Sprinkle flaxseed meal on top and serve.

Green Smoothie Protein Shake

Serves: 1

Ingredients:

- 1 cup fresh spinach leaves
- 5 – 6 drops strawberry extract
- 5 – 6 drops banana extract
- ¼ cup nonfat plain Greek yogurt
- Stevia drops to taste
- 1/3 cup water
- 2 tablespoons vanilla whey protein powder
- Ice cubes, as required

Directions:

1. Add spinach, strawberry extract, banana extract, Greek yogurt, stevia, water, protein powder, and ice cubes into a blender and blend until smooth.
2. Pour into a glass and serve.

Butterfinger Protein Shake

Serves: 2

Ingredients:

- 2 cups ice cubes
- 2 scoops protein powder
- 2 tablespoons sugar-free butterscotch pudding mix
- 2 cups water
- 2 tablespoons natural peanut butter

Directions:

1. Add water, protein powder, peanut butter, ice cubes, and pudding mix into a blender and blend until smooth.

2. Pour into 2 glasses and serve. You can consume one glass of the smoothie and freeze the remaining in ice cube trays or Popsicle molds.

Chapter Six

Gastric Bypass Lunch Recipes

Stage /Phase 1: Clear Liquid Diet (Generally up to 12 – 15 days after surgery, but it can vary)

Chicken Broth

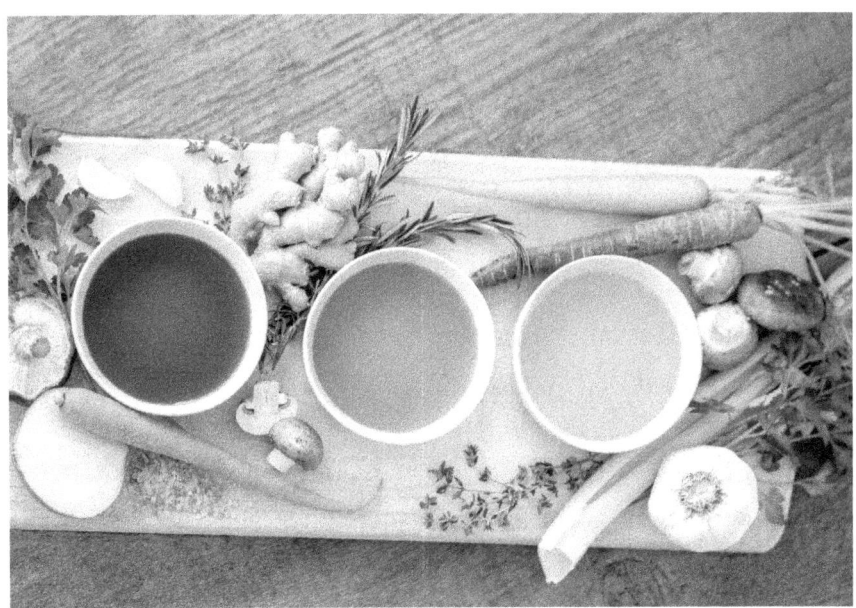

Serves: 10 – 12

Ingredients:

- 4 – 5 pounds chicken, cut into parts
- 8 whole peppercorns
- 8 large carrots, cut into quarters
- 2 large onions, cut into chunks
- 4 tablespoons sea salt
- 5 – 6 bay leaves
- 4 stalks celery, chopped into large pieces
- Water, as required

Directions:

1. Place chicken, peppercorns, carrots, onions, salt, bay leaves, and celery in a large stockpot.

2. Pour about 4 quarts of water. Place the pot over medium heat. When the water starts boiling, turn down the heat to medium heat. Remove the scum that will float on top.

3. Turn the heat to low heat and cook covered for about 2 hours. Add salt to taste.

4. Strain and retain the clear liquids for this phase. Cool completely. Pour it into a container and place it in the refrigerator. Let the stock chill for a couple of hours. Fat will float on top; remove it with any remaining scum and discard it.

5. Heat the stock before serving.

6. For stage 2 and stage 3, discard the skin and bones. Blend the meat and serve

Stage /Phase 2: Liquid and pureed diet (Generally 15 – 30 days after surgery but it can vary)

Creamy Shrimp Scampi Puree

Serves: 2 – 4

Ingredients:

- 1 tablespoon olive oil or water
- 2 cloves garlic
- 1 tablespoon nonfat plain Greek yogurt
- ½ pound shrimp
- 1/8 cup chopped parsley
- A pinch of salt

Directions:

1. Pour water into a pan and let it heat over medium heat. Add garlic and cook for about a minute or until you get a nice fragrance when water is hot.

2. Dry the shrimp by patting it with paper towels and place them in the pan. Spread it evenly and let them cook for a couple of minutes.

3. Turn the shrimp over and cook for a couple of minutes or until the shrimp is cooked and pink.

4. Turn off the heat, and let it cool for a few minutes. Place shrimp in the food processor bowl, add yogurt and blend until smooth.

5. Blend until chunky for stage 3. For stage 4, do not blend the shrimp, simply mix up yogurt and shrimp in a bowl. Add parsley only for this stage.

Turkey Tacos with Refried Beans Puree

Serves: 4

Ingredients:

For the beans:

- ½ clove garlic, peeled, minced
- 1/8 cup low-sodium chicken broth
- ½ cup unsalted cooked or canned pinto beans, rinsed, drained
- 1 tablespoon chopped cilantro
- 1 tablespoon water

For the turkey:

- 1/8 teaspoon mild chili powder
- 1/8 teaspoon paprika
- ¼ pound lean ground turkey
- 1/8 teaspoon garlic powder
- 1/8 teaspoon ground cumin
- 1 tablespoon water or more if required
- A pinch of salt

Directions:

1. Pour water into a pan and let it heat over medium heat. Add garlic and cook for about a minute or until you get a nice fragrance when water is hot.
2. Stir in broth and pinto beans. When the mixture starts boiling, turn down the heat to low heat and cook for 3 to 4 minutes.
3. Mash the beans using a potato masher and cook for about a minute. Turn off the heat.
4. For turkey: Add garlic powder, chili powder, paprika, and cumin into a pan and let it heat over medium-low heat.
5. Keep stirring until you get a nice toasted aroma.
6. Stir in turkey and water. As you stir, crumble the meat. When the water dries up, add another tablespoon of water. Repeat this process until the meat is cooked.
7. Turn off the heat. Cool for 5 – 8 minutes.
8. Transfer the beans and meat into the food processor bowl and process until smooth or the texture you desire is achieved.
9. Transfer into a bowl. Serve small portions of the puree.
10. This can be served in stage 3 as well. Do not blend into a fine puree. Keep it slightly chunky.
11. For the 4th stage, do not blend the turkey and bean mixture; simply mix them up together in a bowl.
12. Add cilantro while mixing up.

Chimichurri Chicken Puree

Serves: 2 – 3

Ingredients:

- ¼ pound lean ground chicken
- 1/8 teaspoon dried oregano
- 1 tablespoon chopped cilantro
- 1 teaspoon apple cider vinegar
- ¼ teaspoon paprika (optional)
- 1/8 cup chopped parsley
- 1 clove garlic, peeled
- 1 tablespoon water + more if required
- Pepper to taste (optional)
- A pinch of salt

Directions:

1. Add water into a skillet and let it heat over medium heat. When water is hot, stir in chicken, oregano, and paprika and stir. As you stir, crumble the meat into smaller pieces.

2. If the chicken is not cooked and there is no liquid in the pan, add another tablespoon of water and cook. Repeat, until the chicken is cooked. Turn off the heat.

3. Blend chicken, salt, oregano, and pepper, if using, in a blender until smooth.

4. Serve. Store leftover puree in an airtight container in the refrigerator. Use it within 4 – 5 days.

5. This puree can be had in stage 3 and stage 4. For stage 3, mix up the chicken, oregano, salt, and pepper. For stage 4, simply mix up the ingredients together. Add parsley and cilantro and mix well.

6. Serve.

Sweet Potato Puree

Serves: 2

Ingredients:

- 1 medium sweet potato, trim the ends
- A pinch of salt
- ¼ teaspoon ground cinnamon
- 3- 5 teaspoons orange juice
- ½ tablespoon half and half or milk
- 1 tablespoon butter
- ¼ teaspoon nutmeg
- 1/8 teaspoon ground black pepper
- Stevia to taste

Directions:

1. Place the sweet potato on parchment paper and wrap it up. Place it in the microwave and cook on high for about 5 minutes or until very soft.

2. Let it cool for 5 minutes. Peel the sweet potato and break it into pieces.

3. For stage 2, place the sweet potato in the blender. Add salt, cinnamon, orange juice, half and half, nutmeg, pepper, and stevia, and blend until smooth.

4. For stage 3, place sweet potato, salt, cinnamon, orange juice, half and half, nutmeg, pepper, and stevia in a bowl and mash until chunky.

5. For stage 4, place sweet potato, salt, cinnamon, orange juice, half and half, nutmeg, pepper, and stevia in a bowl and mix until well combined. Melt butter and add it to the bowl.

6. Mix well and serve.

Chicken and Black Bean Mole Puree

Serves: 4

Ingredients:

- 2 small cloves garlic, minced
- ½ cup unsalted, cooked or canned black beans, rinsed, drained
- 1/8 cup low-sodium chicken broth
- ¼ teaspoon paprika (optional)
- 1/8 teaspoon ground cumin
- 1/8 teaspoon garlic powder
- 1 tablespoon chopped cilantro
- 4 ounces lean ground chicken
- 4 raw almonds, soaked in water for 8 to 9 hours
- ¾ teaspoon raw cacao powder
- 1/8 teaspoon dried oregano
- 1/8 teaspoon ground coriander
- A pinch ground cinnamon
- Water, as required

Directions:

1. Add a tablespoon of water into a pan and let it heat over medium-high heat. Once the water starts steaming, stir in

the garlic. Cook for about a minute or until you get a nice aroma.

2. Stir in the chicken. As you stir, break the chicken into smaller pieces.

3. Add a tablespoon of water whenever the water dries up in the pan. When meat is cooked, turn off the heat. Add black beans and stir.

4. Peel the almonds and add them into a blender. Also add broth, cacao, oregano, coriander, cinnamon, paprika, cumin, and garlic powder and blend until smooth.

5. Add the chicken and black bean mixture and blend until smooth.

6. Serve.

7. Cilantro is to be added while blending, only for stage 3 or 4.

Jell-O Mousse

Serves: 2

Ingredients:

- ½ small box sugar-free Black cherry Jell-O
- 1 container Dannon light and fit cherry Greek yogurt
- ¼ cup warm water
- 1 scoop unflavored protein powder, preferably whey protein powder

Directions:

1. Place Jell-O mix in a bowl. Drizzle warm water over the mix. Allow it to rest for 5 minutes.
2. Add yogurt and protein powder and blend with an immersion blender until smooth.
3. Divide into 2 ramekins and place it at room temperature for it to set.
4. Chill until ready to use.

Stage /Phase 3: Soft diet (Generally between 5 – 12 weeks after surgery but it can vary)

Lentil, Haricot Bean and Chickpea Soup

Serves: 2 – 3

Ingredients:

- 1 tablespoon olive oil + extra to serve if desired
- 2 cloves garlic, peeled, sliced
- 2 cups vegetable stock
- ½ can (from a 15 ounces can) chickpeas, drained, rinsed
- Juice of ½ lemon
- ½ can (from a 15 ounces can) haricot beans, drained, rinsed
- 1 small red bell pepper, finely chopped
- 1 small green bell pepper, finely chopped
- Sea salt to taste
- Freshly ground black pepper to taste
- ½ red onion, finely chopped
- ½ can (from a 14 ounces can) chopped tomatoes
- 2.5 ounces dried red split lentils, rinsed, soaked in water for 30 minutes
- Chopped basil or cilantro to garnish

Directions:

1. Pour oil into a soup pot and let it heat over medium heat.

2. Add onion and garlic when the oil is hot and cook until the onion turns golden brown.

3. Stir in stock, chickpeas, haricot beans, red bell pepper, green bell pepper, salt, pepper, onion, chopped tomatoes, and dried split lentils.

4. The liquid in the pot should cover the ingredients by at least an inch (over the ingredients). Add some water or broth if the liquid does not cover the ingredients.

5. When the mixture starts boiling, turn down the heat to low heat. Add salt and pepper and cook covered for about 20 minutes or until the lentils are cooked. Stir occasionally while cooking.

6. If you find that the lentils are uncooked and no liquid in the pot, feel free to add more broth or water.

7. If your doctor has allowed you to eat chunky food, serve the soup as it is or blend it with an immersion blender until it is smooth or the consistency you desire.

8. Taste the soup. Add more salt and pepper to taste if required.

9. You can add the basil leaves for stage 4.

10. Ladle into soup bowls and serve. If you have any leftover soup, let it cool completely. Pour into an airtight container and place it in the refrigerator until use. You should use it within 4 – 5 days. You can also freeze the leftover soup in a freezer-safe container. It can last for 2 months.

11. Thaw completely. Heat thoroughly in a pan or in the microwave and serve.

Curried Acorn Squash Cream Soup with Coconut Milk

Serves: 4 – 5

Ingredients:

For the squash:

- 2 acorn squashes, halved, deseeded
- ¾ teaspoon kosher salt or to taste
- 1 ½ tablespoons olive oil
- Pepper to taste

For the broth:

- 1 ½ tablespoons coconut oil or butter
- 1 cup chicken stock or vegetable broth
- 2 teaspoons curry powder
- 1 ½ onions, sliced
- 2/3 cup light coconut milk

For roasted acorn squash seeds: Optional

- 8 – 10 tablespoons acorn squash seeds
- ¼ teaspoon onion salt
- ½ teaspoon smoked paprika
- ½ tablespoon olive oil

Directions:

1. Preheat the oven to 400° F.

2. Put the squash halves on a baking sheet, and brush oil on the cut part of the squash.

3. Sprinkle salt and pepper over the cut part of the squash halves.

4. Put the baking dish in the oven and set the timer for 45 minutes or until golden brown on top.

5. Pour oil into a soup pot and place the pot over medium heat. When oil melts, add onion and stir well. Now spread the onions on the bottom of the pot. Do not stir until the underside of the onion is brown. Turn down the heat to medium-low heat.

6. Now give it a good stir and cook for some more time until golden brown. Stir often.

7. Pour in the stock. Scrape the bottom of the pot to remove any browned bits that may be stuck.

8. Remove the peel of the roasted squash and add the pulp into the soup pot.

9. Stir in curry powder. When the soup starts boiling, turn the heat to low heat and cover the pot. Cook for about 15 minutes.

10. Blend with an immersion blender until smooth.

11. Add coconut milk and give it a good stir.

12. This soup is great for the 4th stage as well. Roasted acorn squash seeds are to be served only in stage 4 if desired.

13. To make roasted acorn seeds: Prepare a baking dish by lining it with parchment paper. Remove any flesh if present on the acorn squash seeds.

14. Scatter the acorn squash seeds all over the prepared baking sheet.

15. Place the baking sheet in the oven and set the timer for 15 minutes or until crisp.

16. Let the seeds cool completely. Store the cooled seeds in an airtight container until ready to serve.

17. Serve soup in bowls. Scatter with roasted acorn squash seeds and serve.

Three Bean Turkey Chili

Serves: 4 – 5

Ingredients:

- 1 tablespoon olive oil
- ½ red or yellow bell pepper, chopped
- 3 cloves garlic, peeled, minced
- ½ teaspoon chipotle chili powder
- ½ teaspoon ground coriander
- ¼ teaspoon cayenne pepper
- ½ teaspoon sea salt or to taste
- 1 pound lean ground turkey
- ½ can (from a 15 ounces can) red kidney beans, rinsed, drained
- ½ can (from a 15 ounces can) black beans, rinsed, drained
- ½ can (from a 15 ounces can) white beans, rinsed, drained
- ½ can (from a 14.5 ounces can) tomato puree
- ¼ cup chopped cilantro
- 1 large onion, chopped
- ½ jalapeño chili pepper, deseed if desired, chopped
- 2 tablespoons chili powder or to taste
- ½ tablespoon ground cumin
- ½ teaspoon red pepper flakes

- ¼ teaspoon dried oregano
- ¼ teaspoon freshly ground black pepper
- ½ can (from a 28 ounces can) diced tomatoes
- ½ cup low-sodium chicken broth or water

For toppings: Optional

- ½ fresh jalapeño, deseed if desired, thinly sliced
- Lime wedges
- ½ ripe avocado, peeled, pitted, chopped

Directions:

1. Pour oil into a soup pot or Dutch oven and let it heat over medium heat.
2. Add onion and cook for a couple of minutes when the oil is hot.
3. Stir in bell pepper and jalapeño. Cook for a few minutes until tender, stirring often.
4. Add garlic and stir well. Cook for about a minute or until you get a nice aroma.
5. Stir in chipotle chili powder, chili powder, ground coriander, ground cumin, red pepper flakes, oregano, cayenne pepper, pepper, and salt. Cook until tender.

6. Stir in turkey. As you stir, crumble the meat into smaller pieces.

7. Keep cooking until the meat is not pink anymore. It should take about 8 to 10 minutes. Stir occasionally.

8. Stir in red kidney beans, black beans, white beans, tomato puree, chicken stock, and diced tomatoes.

9. Stir well and cover the pot. When the mixture starts boiling, lower the heat to medium-low heat.

10. Now cover the pot partially and let the mixture simmer for about 25 minutes. Stir the mixture every 10 – 12 minutes.

11. Take a little of the chili and taste it. Add more salt or spices if required. Turn off the heat.

12. Ladle into soup bowls and serve.

13. For stage 4, add cilantro and stir. Garnish with some extra cilantro and jalapeño slices and serve.

Korean Turkey Bowl

Serves: 3

Ingredients:

- 1 tablespoon honey
- 1 teaspoon sesame oil
- 1/8 teaspoon ground ginger
- 2 small cloves garlic, peeled, minced
- 1 green onion, thinly sliced
- 2 tablespoons low-sodium soy sauce
- ¼ teaspoon crushed red pepper flakes or to taste
- ½ tablespoon vegetable oil or olive oil
- ½ pound lean ground turkey
- A pinch sesame seeds
- Sea salt to taste

Directions:

1. Add soy sauce, red pepper flakes, sesame oil, and ginger into a bowl and mix well.

2. Pour oil into a pan and let it heat over medium heat.

3. When the oil is hot, add turkey and cook until brown. As you stir, crumble the meat into smaller pieces. Stir in the sauce mixture. Heat thoroughly. Turn off the heat and serve. Add salt and stir.

4. For stage 4, add honey in step 1. Add the green onion in step 3 while adding the sauce mixture.

5. Garnish with sesame seeds and serve over cauliflower rice.

Creamy White Bean Soup with Kale

Serves: 8 – 10

Ingredients:

- 2 tablespoons olive oil
- 6 stalks celery, diced
- 12 cloves garlic, peeled, finely chopped
- 7 cups low-sodium vegetable broth
- Freshly cracked pepper to taste
- 2 medium Yukon gold potatoes, peeled, finely diced
- 2 cans (14 ounces each) artichoke hearts, drained, rinsed, finely chopped (optional)
- Extra-virgin olive oil to serve (optional)
- ½ large onion, diced
- 1 ½ medium carrots, peeled, diced
- ¼ teaspoon crushed red pepper flakes
- ½ teaspoon kosher salt or more to taste
- 4 cans (15 ounces each) cannellini beans, drained, chopped
- 2 small heads lacinato kale, remove hard ribs, shredded

For bouquet garni:

- 4 bay leaves
- 2 large or 4 small sprigs rosemary
- 2 large sprigs sage

For gremolata:

- 2 cups loosely packed fresh Italian flat-leaf parsley
- 4 large cloves garlic, peeled, grated
- Coarse or flaky sea salt
- 1 cup loosely packed fresh basil leaves
- 3 lemons

Directions:

1. Pour oil into a Dutch oven or soup pot and let it heat over medium-high heat. When the oil is hot, add onion, carrots, and celery and mix well. Add a bit of salt and mix well.

2. Stir often until the onions are light brown. Stir in garlic and red pepper flakes. Cook for a few seconds until you get a nice aroma. Make sure the red pepper flakes do not get burnt.

3. Add broth and stir. Scrape the bottom of the pot to remove any burnt bits that may be stuck.

4. Add salt and pepper to taste.

5. To make bouquet garni: Hold bay leaves, rosemary, and sage together and tie them with kitchen twine.

6. Drop the bouquet garni into the pot. Add potatoes, artichoke hearts, and cannellini beans, and mix well.

7. When the mixture starts boiling, turn down the heat to low heat and cook covered until the potatoes are soft.

8. To make the gremolata: Chop parsley and basil leaves into very fine pieces. Place the herbs in a bowl. Add garlic. Finely grate the lemon peel directly into the bowl.

9. Add flaky sea salt and stir.

10. Turn off the heat. Pour half the soup into a blender. Blend until well pureed. Pour the soup back into the pot.

11. Place the pot over medium heat and stir in the kale. Let the kale cook until it wilts. Do not overcook the kale; it should be bright green in color.

12. Discard the bouquet garni. Taste the soup and add salt and pepper if required.

13. Ladle into soup bowls and serve. Cool the leftover soup completely. Transfer the soup into an airtight container and refrigerate until ready to use.

14. Gremolata is to be served only in stage 4. To serve gremolata, top each bowl with gremolata and extra-virgin olive oil if desired.

Buffalo Ranch Chicken

Serves: 2 – 3

Ingredients:

- 1 can chicken
- 4 ounces low-fat cream cheese
- ¼ cup low-fat Mexican blend shredded cheese
- ¼ cup low-fat sour cream
- ¼ cup Chalula or hot sauce of your choice
- ½ packet ranch seasoning

Directions:

1. Add chicken into the food processor along with its liquid. Add cream cheese, Mexican blend cheese, sour cream, hot sauce, and ranch seasoning and blend until smooth or the texture you desire.

2. You can heat it up in a pan or microwave and serve. Serving cold is not a bad idea.

Stage /Phase 4: Regular diet (Generally after 12 weeks after surgery but it can vary)

Cauliflower Soup

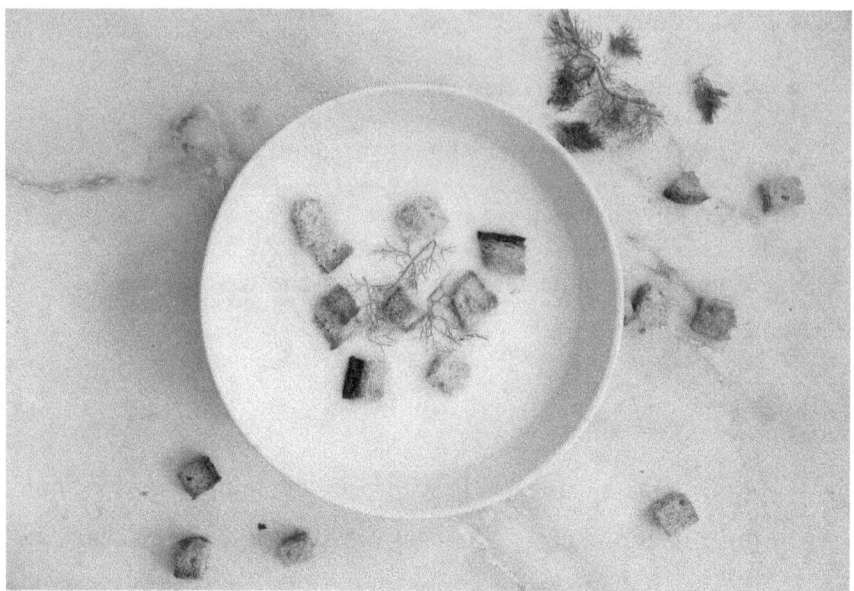

Serves: 3

Ingredients:

- 1 ½ pounds cauliflower florets
- ½ sweet onion, chopped
- 3 ounces low-fat sour cream
- ½ teaspoon seasoned pepper
- Cooked, crumbled bacon to garnish (optional)
- 2 teaspoons minced garlic

- 3 cups chicken broth
- ½ tablespoon coarse ground garlic salt
- ½ jar sun-dried tomatoes
- ½ bunch green onions, finely chopped
- 1 teaspoon Italian seasoning or to taste
- ¼ cup grated reduced-fat parmesan cheese (optional)

Directions:

1. Place a soup pot over medium heat. Spray some cooking spray in the pot.
2. Add onion and garlic and cook until soft.
3. Stir in garlic salt, chicken broth, sun-dried tomatoes, and seasoned pepper.
4. When the mixture starts boiling, turn the heat to low heat and cook covered until the cauliflower is soft. Stir occasionally. Turn off the heat.
5. Blend the soup with an immersion blender until smooth.
6. Stir in sour cream and Parmesan cheese if using. Serve in bowls garnished with bacon and green onions.

Thai Red Curry with Vegetables

Serves: 8

Ingredients:

- 2 ½ cps brown Jasmine rice or long grain brown rice, rinsed well, soaked in water for an hour
- 2 cups chopped onions
- 2 tablespoons finely grated fresh ginger
- 1 bell red bell pepper, deseed if desired, cut into 2-inch long strips
- 1 bell green bell pepper, deseed if desired, cut into 2-inch long strips
- 1 bell yellow bell pepper, deseed if desired, cut into 2-inch long strips
- 1 bell orange bell pepper, deseed if desired, cut into 2-inch long strips
- 4 cloves garlic, pressed or minced
- 2 tablespoons coconut oil or olive oil
- Sea salt to taste
- 4 tablespoons Thai red curry paste
- 1 cup water
- 3 cups packed, thinly sliced kale, discard hard ribs before chopping
- 2 tablespoons soy sauce or tamari

- 3 tablespoons coconut sugar or brown sugar
- 4 teaspoons rice vinegar or fresh lime juice
- ½ can (from a 14 ounces can) regular coconut milk

To serve:

- Chopped fresh cilantro or basil
- Red pepper flakes
- Chili garlic sauce or sriracha (optional)

Directions:

1. To make rice. Boil a large pot of water over high heat. When water starts boiling, drain the water from the soaked rice and add it to the pot. When the water starts boiling again, turn the heat to low heat and cook until the rice is tender.

2. Turn off the heat. Strain the rice in a colander and add it back into the pot. Keep the pot covered until lunchtime.

3. To prepare curry: Pour oil into a large skillet and let it heat over medium heat. When the oil is hot, add onion and a bit of salt and cook until soft and light pink.

4. Stir in ginger and garlic and cook for some seconds until you get a nice aroma.

5. Stir in all the bell peppers and carrots. Cook for a few minutes until the bell peppers are slightly tender.

6. Stir in curry paste. Stir every now and then for about 2 minutes.

7. Stir in sugar, kale, water, and coconut milk. If you can get Tuscan, dinosaur, or lacinato kale, that would be great.

8. When the mixture starts boiling, turn down the heat to medium heat and cook until the vegetables are cooked as per your preference. Make sure to stir the curry occasionally.

9. Turn off the heat. Add rice vinegar, tamari, salt, and pepper. Mix well. Taste the curry and add more tamari, rice vinegar, or salt if necessary.

10. Garnish with cilantro and red pepper flakes and serve.

11. Serve rice and curry. Serve with sriracha sauce if desired.

12. You can store leftover curry and rice in separate airtight containers in the refrigerator. It can last for about 4 days.

Jeweled Rice Pilaf

Serves: 2

Ingredients:

- 2 cups cooked long grain brown rice or wild rice
- ½ bunch scallions, chopped
- 3 tablespoons toasted chopped pistachios
- ¼ cup pomegranate arils
- Sea salt to taste
- 1 teaspoon extra-virgin olive oil
- Freshly ground black pepper to taste
- 2 cloves garlic, peeled, minced
- ¼ cup chopped parsley
- ¼ cup chopped fresh mint leaves
- Roasted chickpeas to serve (optional)

For the dressing:

- 1 tablespoon white wine vinegar
- ½ tablespoon fresh lemon juice
- ¼ teaspoon ground cumin
- 1/8 teaspoon ground cinnamon
- Freshly ground black pepper to taste
- 1 tablespoon extra-virgin olive oil

- ½ tablespoon fresh orange juice
- ½ teaspoon grated orange zest
- ¼ teaspoon maple syrup
- ¼ teaspoon ground coriander
- ¼ teaspoon sea salt

Directions:

1. To make the dressing: Add oil, orange juice, lemon juice, cumin, cinnamon, pepper, vinegar, orange zest, maple syrup, coriander, and salt into a bowl. Whisk well.

2. Cover the bowl and keep it aside for a few minutes for the flavors to blend.

3. Pour oil into a skillet and let it heat over medium heat. When the oil is hot, add garlic, scallions, pepper, and salt and mix well.

4. Cook until scallions are tender.

5. Turn down the heat to low heat. Add rice and mix well. Heat thoroughly. Taste the rice and add more salt and pepper if required. Remember, there is salt in the dressing, so add salt accordingly.

6. Take off the skillet from heat. Pour dressing all over the rice. Scatter pomegranate, parsley, and pistachios on top and give it a good stir. You can taste for salt and pepper once again if desired. Add more if required.

7. Garnish with mint leaves and chickpeas if using and serve.

Roasted Vegetable Pasta

Serves: 2 – 3

Ingredients:

- 2 carrots, trimmed, peeled, cut into 1 inch chunks
- 2 – 3 small patty pan squash, halved
- 5 cherry tomatoes
- ½ tablespoon sherry vinegar
- ¼ teaspoon herbes de Provence
- ½ package (from a 16 ounces package) brown rice penne pasta
- ¼ cup chopped fresh basil + extra to garnish
- Red pepper flakes to taste
- 1 Vidalia onion or ½ small yellow onion, cut into 1-inch pieces
- 1 small zucchini, cut into 1-inch pieces
- ½ tablespoon extra-virgin olive oil + extra to drizzle
- 1 clove garlic, peeled, minced
- 4 sprigs fresh thyme, leaves only + extra to garnish
- 1/8 cup crumbled reduced-fat feta cheese
- Freshly ground black pepper to taste
- 1 tablespoon fresh lemon juice or more to taste
- Sea salt to taste

Directions:

1. Preheat the oven to 400° F.

2. Prepare a large baking sheet by lining it with parchment paper.

3. Scatter the carrots and onion on one side of the baking sheet and drizzle with half the oil. Sprinkle salt and pepper over them and place them in the oven. Set the timer for about 30 minutes or until onions are slightly brown around the edges.

4. Place squash, tomatoes, and zucchini on the other side of the baking sheet. Drizzle half of the remaining oil over these. Sprinkle salt and pepper.

5. Place the baking sheet back in the oven and set the timer for 20 minutes or until the vegetables are tender as well as slightly browned.

6. Take out the baking sheet from the oven.

7. Add sherry vinegar, remaining oil, herbes de Provence, garlic, thyme, pepper, and salt into a bowl and mix well.

8. Add the roasted vegetables and stir well.

9. While the vegetables are roasting, cook the pasta following the directions given on the package of pasta.

10. Drain the pasta and add it to the bowl of roasted vegetables. Mix well.

11. Stir in basil, red pepper flakes, and feta lemon juice. Add salt and pepper to taste. Add some more lemon juice if required. Mix well.

12. Sprinkle some fresh herbs on top. Trickle some olive oil on top and serve.

Greek Pita Sandwiches

Serves: 2

Ingredients:

For dressing:

- 1 tablespoon fresh lemon juice
- 1/8 teaspoon dried oregano
- 1 tablespoon extra-virgin olive oil
- ¼ teaspoon minced garlic
- Sea salt to taste

For pitas:

- 1 whole-wheat pita bread, halved crosswise (this will make 2 pita pockets)
- 1 small cucumber, quartered lengthwise, cut into ¼ inch thick slices crosswise
- ½ tablespoon finely chopped onion
- 3 tablespoon feta cheese or non-dairy cheese (optional)
- Freshly ground pepper to taste
- 1 ¼ cups spinach (cut into ribbons)
- 3 tablespoons pitted, quartered kalamata olives
- ½ cup quartered cherry tomatoes
- 2 – 3 fresh basil leaves, torn
- 6 tablespoons eggplant hummus or regular hummus (optional)

For eggplant hummus:

- ¾ pound eggplant, halved lengthwise
- 1 ½ tablespoons extra-virgin olive oil + extra to drizzle
- 3 tablespoons tahini
- ½ - ¾ teaspoon smoky paprika or regular paprika
- 3 – 5 teaspoons liquid from the can of chickpeas
- 1 can (from a 15 ounces can) chickpeas, drained (but retain 3 – 5 teaspoons of the liquid)
- ¾ teaspoon fine sea salt or to taste
- Juice of ½ lemon
- ½ teaspoon ground cumin
- Zest of ½ lemon, grated
- 2 large cloves garlic, peeled
- Chopped parsley

Directions:

1. To make the dressing: Pour olive oil and lemon juice into a small jar. Add garlic, salt, and oregano and fasten the lid. Shake the jar constantly until well combined.

2. To make the salad: Add cucumber, spinach, onion, olive, feta, tomatoes, and basil into a bowl and toss well.

3. Add pepper to taste and toss once again. Drizzle most of the dressing over the salad and toss well. Taste a bit of the salad and decide if more dressing, salt, or pepper is required.

4. Spread the hummus on the thicker part of the pita bread and fill them with salad.

5. Sprinkle basil over the salad and serve.

6. To make eggplant hummus: Preheat the oven to 400°. Prepare a baking sheet by lining it with parchment paper.

7. Take a piece of foil and place garlic on it. Trickle about ½ teaspoon of oil over the garlic and wrap it loosely.

8. Place it on the baking sheet. Score the eggplant halves on the cut part, and brush oil on the cut part of the eggplant halves.

9. Place the eggplant halves on the baking sheet, with the skin side on top.

10. Place the baking sheet in the oven and set the timer for 30 minutes or until the eggplant halves are cooked. They will shrink in size.

11. Take out the baking sheet and allow it to cool. Peel off the skin and discard it.

12. Place eggplant pulp, chickpeas, garlic, tahini, paprika, cumin, lemon juice, lemon zest, and about 2 to 3 teaspoons

of liquid from the can of chickpeas in the food processor bowl and process until the texture you prefer is achieved. If the hummus is very thick, you can add a teaspoon or 2 of chickpea liquid from the can.

13. Pour into a bowl. Add parsley and some extra-virgin olive oil and stir. You can use regular hummus, homemade or store-bought if you do not want to make this hummus. Use hummus to make the sandwiches.

Tomato Stuffed Roasted Eggplant

Serves: 8

Ingredients:

For eggplants:

- 4 eggplants, halved lengthwise
- Sea salt to taste
- Pepper to taste
- 4 teaspoons olive oil

For the filling:

- 16 ounces red cherry tomatoes, quartered
- 8 tomatillos, cut into eighths
- 16 ounces yellow cherry tomatoes, quartered
- 2 teaspoons dried oregano
- 1 teaspoon chopped fresh thyme
- 4 teaspoons vinegar
- Sea salt to taste
- Pepper to taste
- 2 teaspoons chopped fresh basil
- 4 teaspoons olive oil
- 4 cloves garlic, chopped
- Freshly grated reduced-fat parmesan cheese to serve (optional)

Directions:

1. Preheat the oven to 400° F. Prepare a baking sheet by lining it with aluminum foil.

2. Make cuts on the cut part of the eggplant halves in a crisscross manner, slightly deep but do not go right down up to the skin. Leave about ¼ inch of flesh near the skin.

3. Brush oil over the cut part of the eggplant halves. Season with salt and pepper.

4. Place eggplant halves on the baking sheet and place them in the oven. Set the timer for 30 minutes.

5. Take out the baking sheet from the oven and set it aside to cool.

6. Take a spoon and scoop out the flesh from the eggplants. Make sure to leave ½ inch border all over - these are your eggplant shells. Do not discard the scooped flesh; chop it into small pieces.

7. Add chopped eggplant, tomatoes, tomatillos, oregano, thyme, vinegar, salt, pepper, remaining oil, basil, and garlic into a bowl and mix well.

8. Fill this mixture into the eggplant shells. Top with Parmesan cheese and place it on the baking sheet. Bake for 10 minutes.

9. Serve.

Thai Tofu Quinoa Bowl

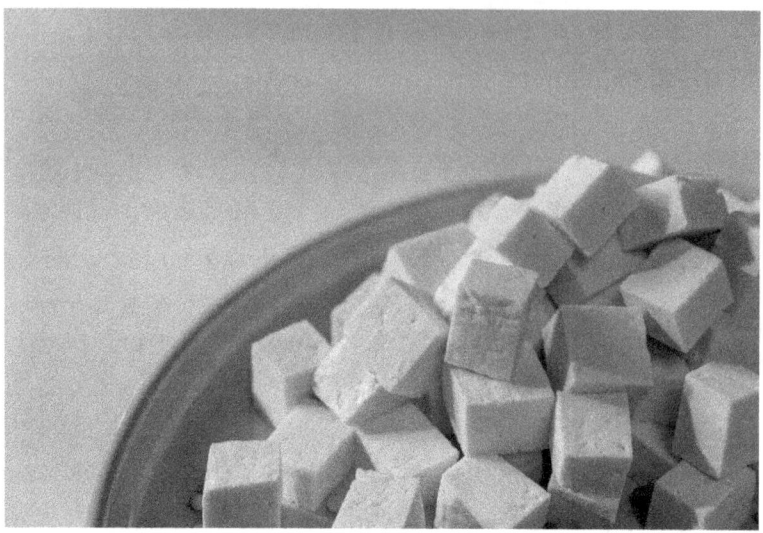

Serves: 3

Ingredients:

- ½ package (from a 15 ounces package) extra-firm tofu, diced
- ½ tablespoon sesame oil
- ¾ cup chicken broth
- ½ cup shredded carrots
- ¼ cup fresh cilantro
- 1 tablespoon soy sauce
- ½ cup uncooked quinoa
- ¼ cup slivered almonds
- 1/3 cup chopped scallions

For the sauce:

- 1 tablespoons sriracha sauce
- 1 ½ tablespoons coconut milk
- 2 small cloves garlic, peeled, minced
- ½ teaspoon grated ginger
- 1 teaspoon creamy peanut butter
- 1 tablespoon rice wine vinegar
- ½ teaspoon brown sugar
- 1 teaspoon lime juice or more to taste

Directions:

1. You need to press the tofu of excess moisture. For this, take the tofu from the package and place it on a plate lined with paper towels. Place something heavy over the tofu, like a cold drink can or heavy pan. Let it remain this way for at least 30 minutes.

2. Preheat the oven to 400° F. Prepare a baking sheet by lining it with aluminum foil or parchment paper.

3. Chop tofu into about 1 inch cubes, and place in a bowl. Pour sesame oil and soy sauce over the tofu and toss well.

4. Spread the tofu on the prepared baking sheet and put it into the oven.

5. Set the timer for about 40 minutes or until brown and crisp all over. Make sure to turn the tofu over every 10 – 12 minutes.

6. Meanwhile, place a pan over medium-low heat. Add quinoa and stir occasionally until quinoa turns golden brown in color.

7. Stir in broth and turn down the heat to low heat. Cook covered until dry. Turn off the heat. Uncover, take a fork and fluff the quinoa grains. Keep it aside.

8. To make the sauce. Melt peanut butter in a microwave-safe bowl in the microwave for 10 seconds.

9. Stir in sriracha sauce, coconut milk, garlic, ginger, rice wine vinegar, brown sugar, and lime juice

10. Add almonds into a small pan and place the pan over low heat. Stir on and off until they are golden brown. Turn off the heat.

11. Add quinoa, almonds, tofu, carrots, cilantro, soy sauce, and scallions into a bowl and mix well.

12. Add sauce mixture and mix well.

13. Serve in bowls.

Tofu and Broccoli Quiche

Serves: 3

Ingredients:

- ¼ cup uncooked bulgur wheat
- ½ cup water
- ½ tablespoon sesame oil
- 4 ounces broccoli florets, chopped
- ¾ pound tofu
- ½ tablespoon white miso or pickled plum paste
- ½ yellow onion, chopped
- 2 ounces mushrooms, chopped
- 1 tablespoon tahini paste
- ½ tablespoon tamari
- Sea salt to taste

Directions:

1. Preheat the oven to 400° F.

2. Pour water into a small saucepan or pot and place it over medium heat.

3. When water starts boiling, add bulgur and a bit of salt. When it starts boiling once again, turn down the heat to low heat and cook covered until dry and tender. If it is uncooked

and there is no water left in the pot, add a couple of tablespoons of water. Turn off the heat.

4. Grease a small pie pan with some cooking spray. Place bulgur in the pie pan and spread it evenly all over the bottom of the pan. Press it well onto the bottom of the pan.

5. Place the pie pan in the oven and set the timer for 12 minutes, or bake until the crust dries up.

6. Pour oil into a skillet and let it heat over medium-high heat. When the oil is hot, add onion, mushrooms, and broccoli and cook for a few minutes until slightly tender.

7. Remove the pan from heat and keep it covered with a lid.

8. Add tahini, tofu, miso, and tamari into a blender and blend until very smooth.

9. Remove the mixture into a bowl. Add onion mixture and mix well. Spread the mixture over the baked crust.

10. Place the pie pan in the oven and set the timer for 30 minutes.

11. Once baked, let it cool for 5 – 8 minutes.

12. Cut into wedges and serve. You can serve this hot or warm or at room temperature.

Black Bean and Brown Rice Casserole

Serves: 4

Ingredients:

- 3 tablespoons brown rice
- ½ tablespoon olive oil
- ½ medium zucchini, thinly sliced
- ¼ cup sliced mushrooms
- 1/8 teaspoon cayenne pepper
- ½ can (from a 4 ounces can) diced green chilies
- 1 cup shredded low-fat Swiss cheese
- ½ cup vegetable broth
- 1 small onion, diced
- 8 ounces cooked, skinless, boneless chicken breast
- ¼ teaspoon ground cumin
- ½ can (from a 15 ounces can) black beans, drained, rinsed
- ¼ cup shredded carrots
- A pinch of salt or to taste

Directions:

1. Add broth and rice into a small pot. Place the pot over medium heat. When the mixture starts boiling, turn the heat to low heat and cook covered until rice is cooked.

2. Preheat the oven to 400° F.

3. Prepare a small casserole dish by spraying it with cooking spray.

4. Pour oil into a skillet and let it heat over medium heat. When the oil is hot, add onion and cook until soft.

5. Add chicken, zucchini, mushrooms, cumin, and cayenne pepper and mix well. Heat thoroughly.

6. Meanwhile, add rice, beans, carrots, chilies, and ½ cup Swiss cheese into a bowl and mix well.

7. Add the chicken mixture and mix well. Spread the mixture into the casserole dish.

8. Scatter remaining Swiss cheese on top. Keep the dish covered loosely with foil.

9. Place the dish in the oven and set the timer for 30 minutes.

10. Remove foil and bake for another 10 minutes or light brown on top.

Jerk Chicken Bowl

Serves: 2 – 3

Ingredients:

For jerk chicken seasoning:

- ½ tablespoon dried thyme
- 1 teaspoon paprika
- ½ teaspoon ground ginger
- ½ teaspoon cayenne pepper
- 1/8 teaspoon pepper
- ½ tablespoon brown sugar
- 1 teaspoon ground all-spice
- ½ teaspoon ground cinnamon
- ½ teaspoon ground cloves
- ½ teaspoon sea salt

For the chicken bowls:

- 2 tablespoons extra-virgin olive oil, divided
- ½ red bell pepper, chopped into 1-inch chunks
- ¼ cup chopped pineapple
- ½ pound chicken breasts
- 2 ½ cups cauliflower rice
- 1 small onion, thinly sliced

- 1/8 cup canned or cooked black beans (optional)
- ½ avocado, peeled, pitted, cut into cubes

Directions:

1. Preheat the oven to 425° F.
2. Add dried thyme, paprika, ginger, cayenne pepper, pepper, brown sugar, all-spice, cinnamon, cloves, and salt into a bowl and stir well.
3. Brush some oil over the chicken. Sprinkle the seasoning mixture over the chicken and massage the seasonings into the chicken.
4. Keep the chicken in a baking dish and bake for about 30 minutes or until the internal temperature of the meat shows 165° F on the meat thermometer.
5. Pour about ½ teaspoon of oil into a pan and let it heat over medium heat. When oil is hot, add cauliflower rice and cook for a couple of minutes.
6. Remove the cauliflower rice into a bowl.
7. Add the remaining oil to the pan. Add onion and bell pepper when the oil is hot and cook until slightly tender.
8. Turn off the heat. Slice the baked chicken.
9. To assemble: Divide cauliflower rice into 2 – 3 bowls. Divide the chicken among the bowls. Place bell pepper and onion mixture over the chicken. Scatter pineapple, black beans, and avocado on top and serve.

Greek Chicken Burgers

Serves: 2

Ingredients:

- ½ pound ground chicken
- 3 tablespoons dried breadcrumbs
- 1 teaspoon dried oregano
- 1/8 cup crumbled reduced-fat feta cheese
- White of a small egg
- ½ teaspoon minced garlic
- Pepper to taste
- ¼ cup coarsely chopped baby spinach
- Sea salt to taste

To serve:

- Whole-wheat or multigrain or gluten-free burger buns
- Lettuce leaves
- Low-fat mayonnaise
- Low-fat cheese of your choice
- Tomato slices
- Salsa
- Guacamole
- Any other toppings of your choice

Directions:

1. Preheat the oven to 500° F. Prepare a baking sheet by lining it with foil.

2. Add chicken, breadcrumbs, oregano, feta, egg white, garlic, pepper, spinach, and salt into a bowl and mix until just combined. Make sure you do not over-mix.

3. Divide the mixture into 2 equal portions and shape into patties.

4. Place them on the baking sheet. Put it in the oven and bake for 15 minutes or until cooked through inside.

5. Serve with suggested serving options if desired.

Tabbouleh and Chicken

Serves: 3

Ingredients:

- ½ cup medium bulgur
- 3 tablespoons olive oil, divided
- ¼ teaspoon garlic powder
- 1 large tomato, deseeded, chopped
- ¼ cup chopped fresh mint
- 2 tablespoons lemon juice
- ¾ cup water
- ½ pound boneless, skinless chicken breast, cut into ½-inch chunks
- Sea salt to taste
- 1 scallion, finely chopped
- ¼ teaspoon garlic powder

Directions:

1. Add bulgur and water into a saucepan and place it over medium heat. When it comes to a boil, turn the heat to low heat and cook covered until tender.

2. Drain the bulgur in a fine wire mesh strainer and rinse with cold water. Drain well and add into a bowl.

3. While the bulgur is cooking, pour a tablespoon of oil into a skillet and let it heat over medium-high heat. When the oil is hot, place the chicken in the pan. Season with salt and garlic powder. Cook until chicken is light brown all over and well-cooked inside. Stir occasionally.

4. Turn off the heat and let the chicken rest for 5 to 8 minutes.

5. Combine scallion, tomatoes, parsley, and mint with bulgur. Add 2 tablespoons of oil, lemon juice, and salt into a small bowl and whisk well. Pour dressing over the bulgur mixture.

6. Mix well. Let it rest for about 30 minutes or longer for the flavors to infuse.

7. Mix well before serving. You can store leftovers in an airtight container in the refrigerator. Use it up within 2 days.

Parmesan Crusted Chicken Tenders

Serves: 2

Ingredients:

- 5 – 6 chicken tenderloins
- ½ tablespoon olive oil
- ¼ cup grated reduced-fat parmesan cheese
- Sea salt to taste
- ¼ cup nonfat Greek yogurt
- Freshly ground pepper to taste
- ¼ cup regular breadcrumbs or Italian flavored panko breadcrumbs

Directions:

1. Preheat the oven to 425° F. Prepare a baking sheet by lining it with foil. Grease the foil with cooking spray.

2. Combine yogurt, oil, salt, and pepper in a shallow bowl.

3. Add breadcrumbs and Parmesan cheese into a shallow bowl and stir.

4. Dip the chicken tenders in yogurt, one at a time. Lift it up and shake off excess yogurt.

5. Next, dredge the chicken in breadcrumbs mixture on one side and place it on the baking sheet with the non-crusted

side facing down and the breadcrumb side facing up. Spray the crumb side with cooking spray.

6. Put it into the oven and set the timer for 8 – 10 minutes or until cooked inside.

7. Set the oven to broil mode and broil for a couple of minutes.

8. Serve immediately.

Thai Chicken Satay with Spicy Peanut Sauce

Serves: 2 – 3

Ingredients:

For chicken satay:

- 1 tablespoon sesame oil
- ½ tablespoon fish sauce
- ½ pound chicken tenders
- Juice of ½ lime
- ½ tablespoon reduced-sodium soy sauce
- ¼ teaspoon chili garlic sauce

For peanut sauce:

- 1 tablespoon light coconut milk
- ½ tablespoon fresh lime juice
- ½ teaspoon brown sugar
- 1 tablespoon smooth natural peanut butter
- ½ tablespoon sesame oil
- ½ tablespoon reduced-sodium soy sauce
- ¼ teaspoon chili garlic sauce

Directions:

1. Set up your grill and preheat it to high heat.

2. Add soy sauce, chili garlic sauce, sesame oil, fish sauce, and lime juice into a bowl and whisk well.

3. Place chicken in the bowl and turn it around in the marinade. Cover and set aside for 15 minutes.

4. Meanwhile, make the peanut sauce: Add coconut milk, peanut butter, lime juice, brown sugar, sesame oil, soy sauce, and brown sugar into a bowl and whisk until well incorporated.

5. If you are using wooden skewers, soak them in water 30 minutes prior to grilling.

6. Fix the chicken tenders on the skewers and lay them on the grill. Turn the skewers every 2 to 3 minutes until the chicken is well-cooked inside.

7. You can serve this hot, warm, or cold with peanut sauce.

Chicken Cordon Bleu Wonton Cupcakes

Serves: 3 (2 cupcakes per serving)

Ingredients:

- 6 ounces cooked, diced chicken breast
- 4 wedges The Laughing Cow Light Swiss Cheese Wedges, chopped
- 12 wonton wrappers
- ¼ cup crushed seasoned croutons
- 1.5 ounces thinly sliced deli ham, chopped
- ½ teaspoon mustard
- 3 slices 2% Swiss cheese, quartered

Directions:

1. Preheat the oven to 425° F. Grease a muffin pan of 6 counts with cooking spray.

2. Add chopped cheese, ham, chicken, and mustard into a microwave-safe bowl and stir.

3. Put it in the microwave and cook on high for about a minute. The cheese would have melted. Mix well. The meat should be coated with cheese.

4. Place a wonton wrapper in each of the muffin cups. The wonton wrapper will more or less take the shape of the muffin cups.

5. Divide equally half the chicken mixture among the muffin cups.

6. Put one piece of Swiss cheese in each cup. Place another wonton wrapper above the Swiss cheese in each cup and press it into the cup.

7. Divide equally the remaining chicken mixture among the cups. Place a piece of Swiss cheese in each.

8. Put the muffin pan in the oven and set the timer for 10 minutes.

9. Scatter crushed croutons on top. Put the muffin pan back into the oven and bake for 8 to 10 minutes or until the wonton wrappers turn golden brown.

10. Let them cool for 5 – 8 minutes before serving.

Chicken Pepper Nachos

Serves: 4 – 5

Ingredients:

- 6 ounces skinless, boneless chicken breast
- 2/3 cup mild salsa
- Low-sodium taco seasoning to taste
- ½ teaspoon chili powder
- ½ teaspoon red pepper flakes
- 1 teaspoon garlic powder
- ½ teaspoon onion powder
- 1 tablespoon lime juice or to taste
- ¾ cup low-fat shredded cheddar and Monterey Jack cheese blend
- A handful of cilantro, chopped
- 1 container (4.4 ounces) fat-free refried beans
- ½ pound mini sweet red bell peppers, trimmed, deseeded, halved lengthwise
- 1/8 cup sliced olives

<u>To serve:</u> Optional

- Low-fat sour cream
- Salsa
- Guacamole

Directions:

1. If you have a crock pot, make this in it or use a heavy pan.

2. Spread the chicken on the bottom of the pan or pot. Add salsa and refried beans over the chicken. Mix well.

3. Combine taco seasoning, onion powder, garlic powder, red pepper flakes, garlic powder, and chili powder in a bowl. Sprinkle it over the salsa and refried beans.

4. Give it a good stir. If you are cooking in a crock pot, set the pot on 'Low' and timer for 5 – 6 hours. If you are cooking on your stovetop, cook on medium-low heat until the chicken is cooked.

5. Once the chicken is cooked, take a pair of forks and shred the chicken.

6. Preheat the oven to 400° F. Prepare a baking sheet by lining it with foil.

7. Press each bell pepper piece to make it flat and place it on the baking sheet.

8. Top each bell pepper piece with some chicken mixture. Scatter cheese on top of the chicken. Place olive slices all over. Place the baking sheet in the oven and set the timer for 10 minutes or until the cheese melts.

9. Drizzle lime juice on top. Garnish with cilantro and serve with suggested serving options.

Mexican Chicken Quinoa Salad Wraps

Serves: 2 – 3

Ingredients:

For the filling:

- ½ pound chicken breasts
- ½ teaspoon ground cumin
- ¼ teaspoon onion powder
- 1/8 teaspoon pepper
- ½ teaspoon chili powder
- ¼ teaspoon garlic powder
- 1/8 teaspoon sea salt
- Olive oil, as required
- ½ can (from a 15 ounces can) black beans, drained, rinsed
- ¼ cup diced cherry tomatoes
- ½ avocado, peeled, pitted, diced
- ½ tablespoon olive oil
- ½ cup fresh or frozen corn
- ½ cup cooked quinoa
- 1 scallion, thinly sliced

For the dressing:

- 2/3 cup nonfat plain Greek yogurt

- 2 – 3 tablespoons finely chopped cilantro
- Pepper to taste
- Juice of ½ lime
- Sea salt to taste

For the wraps:

- Low-carb tortillas or sprouted grain tortillas or whole-wheat tortillas or large lettuce leaves
- A large handful of fresh greens of your choice like spinach or arugula etc.
- Hummus, as required

Directions:

1. Combine cumin, onion powder, garlic powder, pepper, chili powder, and salt in a bowl.
2. Sprinkle this mixture all over the chicken and place it on a plate.
3. Pour oil into a skillet and let it heat over medium heat. When the oil is hot, place the chicken in the pan and cook for about 4 to 5 minutes. Flip the chicken over and cook the other side for 4 to 5 minutes or until well-cooked inside.
4. Turn off the heat. Remove chicken from the skillet and place it on your cutting board. When it cools slightly, cut into bite-size pieces.

5. Meanwhile, prepare the dressing by whisking together yogurt, cilantro, pepper, salt, and lime juice in a bowl. Cover the bowl and let it rest for a few minutes for the flavors to meld.

6. Add chicken, scallions, cherry tomatoes, corn, black beans, and quinoa into a bowl and mix well. You can cook quinoa following the directions given on the package of quinoa. You can also use leftover quinoa if you have any. Add some lime juice if desired.

7. Add avocado and fold gently. Add dressing and toss gently until well incorporated.

8. To assemble the wraps: Spread wraps on serving plates. Spread some hummus on each wrap. Scatter greens. Place chicken mixture on the bottom third of each wrap. Roll them up tightly and place with the seam side facing down.

9. Fasten with toothpicks.

10. Serve.

Chicken Tetrazzini

Serves: 3

Ingredients:

- ½ tablespoon low-calorie margarine
- 4 ounces button mushrooms, sliced
- 1/8 teaspoon garlic powder
- ½ cup fat-free chicken broth
- 4 ounces chicken breasts, skinless, boneless, cubed
- 1 tablespoon sherry cooking wine
- 4 ounces whole-wheat or gluten-free spaghetti, broken into thirds
- ¼ cup chopped scallions
- 1 ½ tablespoons all-purpose flour
- Black pepper or to taste
- ¼ cup fat-free skim milk
- 1/8 cup canned pimentos, drained, sliced
- 1/8 cup reduced-fat parmesan cheese, grated
- Sea salt to taste

Directions:

1. Follow the directions given on the package of spaghetti and cook the spaghetti. Drain and set it aside.

2. Add margarine into a saucepan and place it over medium-high heat. When margarine melts, add scallions and mushrooms and cook for 5 – 6 minutes.

3. Add flour, pepper, milk, garlic powder, salt, and broth into a bowl and whisk until well combined.

4. Pour the mixture into the saucepan. Stir constantly until the mixture thickens.

5. Add pimentos, chicken and sherry. Heat thoroughly. Stir on and off.

6. Add cheese and spaghetti and fold in gently.

7. Serve hot.

Asian Chicken Lettuce Wraps

Serves: 2

Ingredients:

- ½ can (from an 8 ounces can) bamboo shoots, drained, minced
- 1 ½ tablespoons sherry wine
- ½ tablespoon unsalted peanut butter
- ½ teaspoon honey or sugar-substitute to taste
- ½ cup minced onion
- ½ tablespoon minced fresh ginger
- ¼ pound ground chicken breast
- Sea salt to taste
- Bibb or iceberg lettuce leaves to serve
- ½ can (from an 8 ounces can) water chestnuts, drained, minced
- 1 tablespoon hoisin sauce or to taste
- ½ tablespoon soy sauce
- ½ tablespoon minced garlic
- ½ teaspoon sesame oil
- 1 teaspoon sriracha sauce (optional)

To serve:

- ½ small cucumber, deseeded, cut into 1-inch strips

- ½ medium carrot, shredded (optional)
- ½ cup sliced green onions (white and green parts)
- ¼ cup red cabbage (optional)

Directions:

1. Add hoisin sauce, sriracha, sesame oil, sherry, peanut butter, honey, and soy sauce into a bowl Whisk until smooth.

2. Add water chestnuts and bamboo shoots and stir until well combined. Keep it aside.

3. Heat a pan over medium-high heat. When the pan is hot, spray the pan with cooking spray. Add onion and cook until pink. Stir in the garlic and cook for about a minute or until you get a nice aroma. Stir in ginger, ground chicken, and salt. As you stir, make sure to break the meat.

4. Drain off fat, if any, from the meat and move the meat to the edge of the pan.

5. Add sauce mixture with bamboo shoots and water chestnuts and mix well. Heat thoroughly. Turn off the heat.

6. Place lettuce leaves on a large serving platter. Divide the meat mixture among the leaves. Garnish with green onions, carrots, and cucumber and serve.

7. Ground chicken in the recipe can be swapped with lean ground turkey or lean ground beef.

Mediterranean Chicken Wraps

Serves: 3 – 4

Ingredients:

- 1/8 cup nonfat plain Greek yogurt
- ½ teaspoon herbes de Provence
- 1/8 cup julienne cut sun-dried tomatoes packed in oil
- 1/8 cup sliced black olives
- 1 clove garlic, minced
- 4 corn and wheat blend tortillas (6 inches each)
- 1 cup chopped spinach
- 1/8 cup low-fat cream cheese
- ¼ teaspoon sea salt
- 1/8 cup crumbled reduced-fat feta cheese
- 1/8 cup diced cucumber
- 1 tablespoon chopped fresh basil
- ½ pound diced cucumber, peeled, deseeded

Directions:

1. Add cream cheese, Greek yogurt, salt, and herbes de Provence into a bowl and mix well. Cover and keep it aside for about 10 minutes for the flavors to blend.

2. Add feta cheese, sun-dried tomatoes, olives, basil, garlic, and cucumber into a bowl and mix well.

3. Take about a tablespoonful of the cream cheese mixture and spread it on each of the tortillas.

4. Scatter the sun-dried tomato mixture, spinach, and chicken over the tortillas.

5. Roll the tortillas and place with their seam side facing down. Cut into 2 halves if desired.

6. Serve wraps with some fresh fruit like berries or peach or pear.

Chicken Chile Verde

Serves: 2

Ingredients:

- 1 Anaheim peppers, deseeded, remove membranes or ribs
- 1 Serrano pepper, deseeded, remove membrane or ribs
- 2 small white onions, cut into round slices
- 1 boneless, skinless chicken thigh
- 1 boneless, skinless chicken breast
- 2 cups chopped cilantro + extra to garnish
- ½ tablespoon ground cumin
- ¼ teaspoon pepper or to taste
- ¾ cup water
- ½ tablespoon minced garlic
- 2 cups chicken broth
- 3 tomatillos, quartered
- Sea salt to taste
- Maggie seasoning to taste (optional)
- ¼ red onion, thinly sliced, to garnish
- ½ tablespoon ground cumin
- ¼ teaspoon ground pepper
- ¾ cup water

Directions:

1. Combine chicken, pepper, tomatillos, white onion, Serrano peppers, and garlic in a skillet.

2. Sprinkle salt, cumin, pepper, and Maggie seasoning over the mixture and mix well.

3. Add broth and stir. Place the skillet over high heat.

4. When the mixture starts boiling, turn the heat to low heat and simmer until the chicken is cooked.

5. Fish out the chicken from the skillet and place it on a plate. Shred the chicken with a pair of forks.

6. Blend the ingredients in the skillet using an immersion blender until smooth.

7. Add the chicken back into the skillet.

8. Combine cilantro and a little water in a bowl and blend with an immersion blender until smooth. Pour blended cilantro into the skillet.

9. Garnish with cilantro and red onion and serve.

Sour Cream Chicken Enchiladas

Serves: 3

Ingredients:

- 2 tablespoons butter
- 1 ½ cups chicken broth
- A large pinch chipotle chili powder
- 3 ounces chopped green chilies
- 2/3 cup low-fat sour cream
- 4 teaspoons water
- ¼ teaspoon kosher salt or to taste
- 1/3 teaspoon dried oregano
- 2 whole boneless, skinless chicken breast halves
- 1 ½ cups reduced-fat Colby Jack cheese
- 2 cups frozen cauliflower rice
- 2 tablespoons flour or 2 teaspoons arrowroot powder or 1 tablespoon cornstarch

Directions:

1. Melt butter in a skillet over medium heat.
2. Meanwhile, combine flour, arrowroot powder, or cornstarch with 4 teaspoons of cold water and pour into the skillet.

3. Pour broth, stirring constantly. Stir continuously until thick. Add chipotle chili, salt, green chilies, and oregano and mix well. Lay the chicken in the skillet. When it starts boiling, turn down the heat to low heat. Cook covered until chicken is well-cooked.

4. Remove chicken from the skillet with a slotted spoon and place on a plate.

5. Shred the chicken with a pair of forks and add it back into the skillet.

6. Also add in the sour cream and frozen cauliflower rice. Mix well.

7. Cook covered until cauliflower is tender, about 5 to 7 minutes.

8. Sprinkle cheese on top. Cover and cook for a couple of minutes until the cheese melts.

Zucchini Noodles with Turkey Marinara

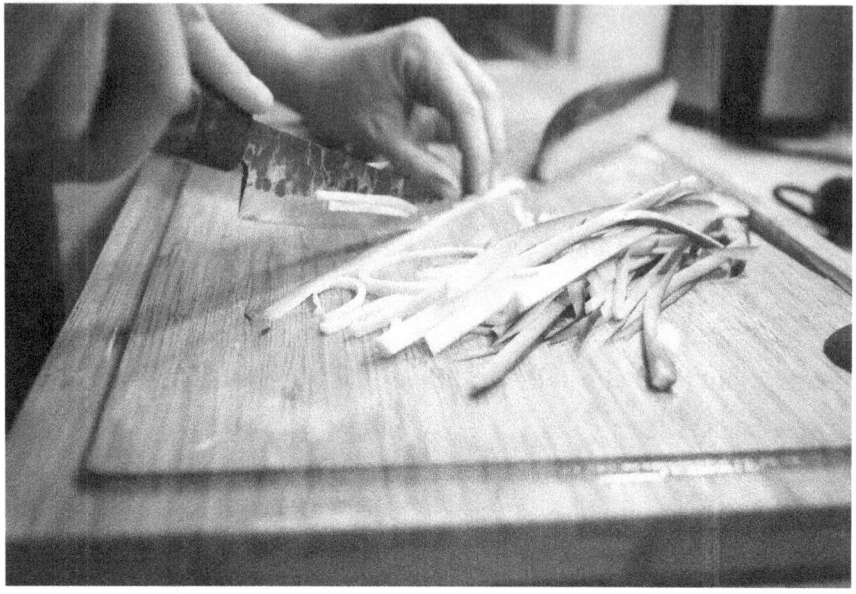

Serves: 2

Ingredients:

For zucchini noodles:

- ½ tablespoon olive oil
- 1 – 2 medium zucchini, trimmed

For turkey marinara sauce:

- ½ pound ground lean turkey
- ½ teaspoon minced garlic
- ½ medium onion, minced
- 1/8 teaspoon dried thyme

- ½ teaspoon Worcestershire sauce
- ¼ teaspoon sugar
- Freshly cracked pepper to taste
- 1 tablespoon olive oil
- ½ can (from a 28 ounces can) tomato sauce or crushed tomatoes or diced tomatoes
- ¼ teaspoon paprika
- ¼ teaspoon ground dry mustard
- Sea salt to taste
- ¼ cup grated, reduced-fat parmesan cheese

Directions:

1. Make zucchini noodles using a spiralizer. You can also use a julienne peeler to make the noodles.
2. Pour ½ tablespoon of oil into a saucepan and let it heat over medium-high heat.
3. Add zucchini noodles when the oil is hot and cook for a few minutes until tender.
4. Transfer onto a plate.
5. To make turkey marinara sauce: Pour ½ tablespoon of oil into the skillet and let it heat.

6. Now add onion and garlic and cook until the onion turns soft. Stir now and then.

7. Stir in turkey. As you stir, crumble the meat. Once the turkey is light brown in color, stir in thyme, tomato sauce, paprika, dry mustard, salt, sugar, pepper, and Worcestershire sauce.

8. When the mixture starts bubbling, turn the heat to low heat and cook for about 15 – 20 minutes until thick. Stir every now and then. Turn off the heat.

9. To assemble: Place zucchini noodles on individual serving plates.

10. Spoon turkey marinara sauce over the noodles. Garnish with Parmesan cheese and serve.

Fajita Turkey Burger

Serves: 8

Ingredients:

- 2 pounds lean ground turkey
- 1 cup grated reduced-fat parmesan cheese
- 1 teaspoon pepper or to taste
- 2 medium onions, sliced
- 1 red bell pepper, sliced
- 1 orange bell pepper, sliced
- 1 green bell pepper, sliced
- 1 orange bell pepper, sliced
- 2 egg whites
- 1 teaspoon salt or to taste
- 4 tablespoons taco seasoning or to taste

Serving options:

- Salsa
- Guacamole
- Low-fat mayonnaise
- Whole-wheat burger buns or lettuce leaves or low-carb buns
- Tomato slices
- Lettuce leaves

Directions:

1. Add ground turkey, egg whites, 2 tablespoons taco seasoning, Parmesan cheese, pepper, and salt into a bowl and mix well. Make sure you do not over-mix; else, the meat will become tough.

2. Make 8 equal portions of the mixture and shape them into patties.

3. Set up a grill and preheat it to medium heat. Grease the grill grate with some oil.

4. Place the burgers on the grill and cook for 4 to 5 minutes. Turn the burgers over and cook the other side for 4 to 5 minutes or until the internal temperature of the meat shows 165° F on the meat thermometer.

5. While the burgers are cooking, place a skillet over medium-high heat. Spray the pan with cooking spray.

6. Add onions and all the bell peppers and cook for 3 to 4 minutes.

7. Stir in remaining taco seasoning and mix well. Cook for a couple of minutes. Turn off the heat.

8. Serve bell pepper mixture over burgers with any one or more of the suggested serving options.

Moroccan Turkey Meatballs

Serves: 8

Ingredients:

For the meatballs:

- 2 pounds ground turkey
- ½ teaspoon finely grated fresh ginger
- 1 teaspoon ground allspice
- ½ teaspoon ground cinnamon
- 2 teaspoons ground cumin
- 2 teaspoons ground coriander
- 1 teaspoon garlic powder
- ½ cup finely chopped fresh parsley
- 1 cup plain whole-wheat breadcrumbs
- Pepper to taste
- 2 large eggs
- Salt to taste
- Oil to cook the meatballs

For the sauce:

- 2 cans (15 ounces each) tomato sauce
- 1 teaspoon sweet paprika
- Red pepper flakes to taste

- Pepper to taste
- 1/8 teaspoon ground cumin
- Sea salt to taste
- Chopped cilantro to garnish

To serve:

- Cauliflower rice
- Brown rice

Directions:

1. To make meatballs: Firstly, prepare a large baking sheet by lining it with parchment paper.

2. Mix together ground turkey, eggs, ginger, breadcrumbs, parsley, allspice, cumin, coriander, garlic powder, parsley, pepper, and salt in a bowl. Mix until just combined, making sure not to over-mix.

3. Dust your hands with some flour and make meatballs of the desired size of the mixture.

4. Place the meatballs on the prepared baking sheet. You can use as many as required and freeze the remaining if desired. For freezing, you can put them in freezer-safe containers or bags.

5. Just in case you are making only a few, keep them in the refrigerator for 10 minutes.

6. Pour oil into a skillet and let it heat over medium-high heat. When oil is hot, add meatballs into the skillet and cook until brown all over. Stir on and off.

7. Remove meatballs with a slotted spoon and place them on a plate lined with paper towels.

8. To make the sauce: Combine tomato sauce, sweet paprika, red pepper flakes, pepper, cumin, and salt in a saucepan.

9. Place the saucepan over medium-low heat. When the mixture starts simmering, it is time to add the meatballs.

10. Drop the meatballs in the sauce and heat thoroughly.

11. If you are freezing some meatballs, don't forget to cool some of the sauce and freeze that too, in freezer-safe containers or bags. Pour into freezer-safe containers or bags and freeze until further use.

12. Garnish with cilantro and serve with suggested serving options.

Turkey Meatloaf

Serves: 8

Ingredients:

- 2 pounds lean ground turkey (about 93% lean)
- 1 medium onion, finely chopped
- 4 teaspoons Worcestershire sauce
- 2 teaspoons cayenne or red pepper or pepper
- 2 teaspoons paprika
- 2 tablespoons garlic powder
- Sea salt to taste
- 2 large eggs
- 2 cups chopped red pepper
- ½ cup grated reduced-fat parmesan cheese
- 2 tablespoons onion powder
- 2 tablespoons low-carb or low-sugar ketchup (optional)
- 2 teaspoons black pepper

Directions:

1. Preheat the oven to 400° F.
2. Combine ground turkey, peppers, and onions in a large bowl.

3. Sprinkle cayenne pepper, onion powder, salt, paprika, garlic powder, and pepper over the mixture and mix well using your hands or a large spoon until just combined.

4. Mix in the eggs and Worcestershire sauce. Next add the Parmesan cheese and mix. Do not over-mix; else, the meat will become tough.

5. Place the meat mixture in a loaf pan of about 9 x 5 inches and keep it on a baking sheet.

6. Place the baking sheet in the oven and set the timer for 40 to 45 minutes.

7. Spread ketchup on the meatloaf 5 minutes before the timer goes off.

8. Let it cool for about 15 – 20 minutes on your countertop.

9. Slice and serve. Store leftover meatloaf slices in an airtight container in the refrigerator. You can also put them in freezer-safe bags and freeze until ready to use. It can last for 4 – 6 weeks.

10. Reheat in a microwave for a few seconds and serve.

Turkey Tagine with Fruit and Nut Couscous and Yogurt Dip

Serves: 2

Ingredients:

For turkey tagine:

- ¾ pound dark turkey or chicken meat from leg or thigh parts
- ¼ cup white wine
- 6 red pearl onions or shallots, peeled, halved
- 1 tablespoon olive oil, divided
- ½ cup chicken stock
- 1 clove garlic, peeled, crushed
- 1 clove garlic, minced
- ¼ teaspoon fennel seeds
- 2 small bay leaves
- ¼ teaspoon ground cumin
- ¼ teaspoon ground ginger
- ½ tablespoon ground coriander
- ¼ teaspoon freshly ground black pepper or to taste
- 2 whole cloves
- ½ inch fresh ginger, peeled
- Freshly ground pepper to taste
- ½ inch stick cinnamon

- ¼ cup capers
- 1/8 cup sliced almonds
- 1/8 cup ground almonds
- 1/8 cup golden raisins (optional)
- 1 tablespoon chopped cilantro root
- Chopped fresh cilantro to garnish
- Zest of ½ lemon, finely grated
- Sea salt to taste

For fruit and nut couscous:

- ½ cup whole-wheat couscous
- 3 tablespoons toasted pine nuts
- 1 tablespoon raisins
- 2 dried apricots, chopped
- ¾ cup water
- 2 tablespoons olive oil
- 2 small cloves garlic, minced
- 1 tablespoon white wine vinegar
- Pepper to taste
- ¾ teaspoon ground cinnamon
- Sea salt to taste
- Juice of ½ lemon

- ¼ cup sliced, toasted almonds
- 2 small green onions, sliced
- 1/8 cup chopped fresh mint leaves
- 1/8 cup chopped fresh cilantro leaves

For yogurt dip:

- ½ cup plain, nonfat yogurt
- ½ tablespoon honey
- 1 tablespoon minced cilantro

Directions:

1. Preheat the oven to 400° F.
2. To make turkey tagine: Add minced garlic, cumin, ginger, coriander, and pepper into a bowl and stir. Stir in the turkey pieces. Stir well so that the turkey pieces are well coated with the spice mixture.
3. Pour ½ tablespoon oil into a skillet. Add turkey and cook until brown all over when the oil is hot.
4. Stir in white wine. Scrape the bottom of the pot to remove any browned bits that may be stuck.
5. Let it boil down to half its original quantity.
6. Stir in stock and cook for 3 – 4 minutes. Turn off the heat.

7. Pour the remaining oil into a tagine (earthen cookware) or an ovenproof skillet (with a fitting lid) and let it heat over medium heat. When oil is hot, add onions and crushed garlic and cook until light brown.

8. Stir in fennel seeds, cloves, ginger, cinnamon, and bay leaves.

9. Keep stirring for about a minute or until the spices are lightly toasted and you have a nice aroma.

10. Add capers and raisins if using. Stir in all the almonds, ground and sliced.

11. Add turkey and stir. When the mixture starts simmering, stir in cilantro roots and lemon zest.

12. Turn off the heat. Add salt to taste and stir.

13. Close the lid and shift the tagine into the oven. Set the timer for about 30 minutes or cook until the turkey is well-cooked.

14. Sprinkle cilantro leaves on top.

15. To make yogurt dip: Combine yogurt, honey, and cilantro in a bowl. Cover and set aside until the couscous is prepared.

16. To make couscous, boil water in a saucepan and add raisins and apricots. Let it boil for 2 minutes and turn off the heat.

17. Place couscous in a bowl. Pour the boiled water, including apricots and raisins, over the couscous. Cover the bowl and let it rest for 10 minutes

18. Take a fork and fluff the couscous grains. Let it cool completely.

19. Add green onions, almonds, cilantro, pine nuts, and mint, and stir.

20. Add oil, garlic, lemon juice, white wine vinegar, and cinnamon to a bowl. Whisk well. Add salt and pepper to taste.

21. Pour this mixture over the couscous. Toss well.

22. Serve turkey tagine with yogurt dip and fruit and nut couscous.

Ground Beef and Vegetable Stew

Serves: 4

Ingredients:

- ½ pound lean ground beef (90% lean)
- 2 small cloves garlic, peeled, finely chopped
- 1 tablespoon beef base
- ½ tablespoon Worcestershire sauce
- ¼ teaspoon celery salt
- 2 – 3 large carrots, cut into round slices
- 8 – 10 green beans, cut into 1-inch pieces
- 1 tablespoon water or more if required
- ½ small onion, finely chopped
- 2 cups water
- ½ can (from an 8 ounces can) tomato sauce
- ½ teaspoon ground black pepper
- 1/8 teaspoon ground marjoram
- 2 medium potatoes, peeled, cut into cubes
- 1 ½ tablespoons all-purpose flour

Directions:

1. Place a skillet over medium-high heat. Add beef, garlic, and onion when the pan is hot and cook until brown.

2. As you stir, crumble the meat into smaller pieces. Discard any cooked fat from the skillet.

3. Stir in beef base and water. Stir in tomato sauce, pepper, marjoram, Worcestershire sauce, and celery salt.

4. When it starts simmering, turn down the heat to low heat.

5. Stir in the carrots and potatoes and cook covered for about 30 minutes. Stir occasionally. Add green beans and stir. When green beans are tender, check the thickness of the stew. If there is more liquid in the skillet, combine flour with a little water and pour it into the skillet. Stir constantly until thick.

6. Let it cook for a few minutes and serve.

7. Store leftover stew after cooling in an airtight container. Reheat the stew and serve.

8. You can serve the stew with low-carb bread, over cauliflower rice, or brown rice.

Pizza Casserole

Serves: 4

Ingredients:

- 7 ounces cauliflower florets, cut into bite-size pieces
- 1 pound Italian sausage, remove casing is present
- 4 ounces mushrooms, cut into slices
- 6 ounces mozzarella cheese, shredded
- 1/8 cup powdered reduced-fat parmesan cheese
- 1.25 ounces pepperoni
- ½ tablespoon olive oil
- ½ green bell pepper, cut into 1-inch squares
- ¾ cup low-carb pasta sauce
- ½ teaspoon Italian seasoning

Directions:

1. Put the cauliflower florets into a microwave-safe container and pour about a cup of water in the bowl.
2. Cover the bowl with a moist paper towel and place it in the microwave. Cook on High for 3 minutes or until the cauliflower is tender. Make sure you do not overcook the cauliflower.
3. Drain off the cauliflower in a colander. Let it sit for 5 minutes.

4. Now dry the cauliflower florets by patting them with paper towels.

5. Preheat the oven to 400° F.

6. Add Italian sausage into a skillet and place it over medium-high heat. Cook until brown. As you stir, crumble the meat into smaller pieces.

7. Transfer the meat into a bowl. Add oil into the skillet. When oil is hot, add mushrooms. Raise the heat to medium-high heat and cook until tender. Turn off the heat.

8. Add cauliflower, mushrooms, and bell peppers into the bowl of sausage and mix well.

9. Spoon half the mixture into a small casserole dish and spread it evenly. Spread ¼ cup of pasta sauce over the meat mixture.

10. Next, spread one-third of the pepperonis, followed by half the mozzarella cheese.

11. Repeat these layers once again.

12. Spread the remaining pasta sauce on top. Add Italian seasoning and Parmesan cheese into a bowl and mix well.

13. Scatter this mixture over the pasta sauce layer. Place remaining pepperoni slices on top and put the casserole dish in the oven.

14. Set the timer for 30 minutes or until the cheese melts and is browned in a few places.

Bacon Cheeseburger Casserole

Serves: 4 – 5

Ingredients:

- 3 ounces bacon
- ¾ pound lean ground beef
- ½ teaspoon dried parsley
- ½ teaspoon sea salt or to taste
- 10 ounces frozen cauliflower rice
- ½ tablespoon avocado oil or any cooking oil
- ½ teaspoon onion powder
- ½ teaspoon garlic powder
- ¼ teaspoon pepper or to taste
- 3 tablespoons coconut flour
- 4 ounces cheddar cheese

For the sauce:

- ½ tablespoon coconut flour
- 1 tablespoon mustard
- ½ tablespoon butter or margarine
- ¾ cup low-fat cream

Directions:

1. Preheat the oven to 400° F.

2. Spread the bacon slices on a baking sheet. Place the baking sheet in the oven and set the timer for 20 minutes or until the bacon is crispy.

3. Take out the baking sheet and let it cool. Chop into pieces.

4. Pour oil into a skillet and let it heat over medium heat. When the oil is hot, add beef and cook until brown.

5. Add parsley, onion powder, garlic powder, pepper, and salt and mix well.

6. Cook for a couple of minutes. Using a slotted spoon, take out the mixture and place in a bowl. Cover the bowl.

7. Add cauliflower into a microwave-safe bowl and place it in the microwave. Cook on high for about 4 minutes or until tender.

8. Stir in salt and coconut flour.

9. To prepare the sauce: Melt the butter in a skillet over medium heat. Add coconut flour and keep stirring until a roux is formed.

10. Add cream and mustard and keep stirring until the sauce is thick. Turn off the heat.

11. To assemble: Pour about ¼ cup of sauce into a baking dish of about 6 – 8 inches.

12. Spread it all over the bottom of the dish.

13. Scatter cauliflower mixture over the sauce layer. Spread it evenly.

14. Next sprinkle half the cheddar cheese over the cauliflower, then layer with ground beef.

15. Next spread half of the sauce that is left. Sprinkle remaining cheddar cheese on top.

16. Now spread the remaining sauce over the cheddar cheese, and scatter bacon on top.

17. Cover the baking dish with foil and put it into the oven.

18. Set the timer for 25 – 30 minutes. Remove the foil and continue baking for a few minutes.

Easy Beef Chili

Serves: 4

Ingredients:

- 1 tablespoon olive oil
- 1 pound lean ground beef (90% lean)
- 2 cloves garlic, peeled, minced
- ½ jalapeño pepper, deseeded, diced
- ½ tablespoon brown sugar (optional)
- 1 teaspoon hot sauce or to taste
- ½ beef bouillon cube, crumbled
- ½ can (from a 14.5 ounces can) diced tomatoes, with its liquid
- ½ onion, diced
- Sea salt to taste
- ½ green bell pepper, deseeded, diced
- Pepper to taste
- ½ green bell pepper, deseeded, diced
- 1 ½ tablespoons tomato paste
- 1 teaspoon Worcestershire sauce
- ½ cup chicken broth
- ½ can (from a 28 ounces can) crushed tomatoes
- ½ can (from a 15 ounces can) kidney beans, drained

- ½ teaspoon ground cumin
- ½ teaspoon mustard powder
- ½ teaspoon dried oregano
- 1/8 teaspoon red pepper flakes
- 1 ¼ tablespoons chili powder
- 1/8 teaspoon cayenne pepper

To serve: Optional

- Low-fat sour cream
- Shredded low-fat cheddar cheese
- Lime wedges
- Tortilla chips

Directions:

1. Pour oil into a soup pot or Dutch oven. Place the pot over medium heat. When the oil is hot, add onion and cook until translucent and soft as well.

2. Stir in ground beef. Raise the heat to medium-high heat. Cook until the meat is not pink anymore. As you stir, crumble the meat.

3. Stir in garlic, jalapeño pepper, and bell pepper. Stir often for about 3 minutes.

4. Add ground cumin, mustard powder, dried oregano, red pepper flakes, chili powder, and cayenne pepper.

5. Cook for a few seconds until you get a nice aroma.

6. Stir in brown sugar, hot sauce, Worcestershire sauce, and tomato paste.

7. Stir well for about a minute. Stir in broth. Scrape the bottom of the pot to remove any browned bits that may be stuck.

8. Sprinkle beef bouillon cubes over the mixture. Give it a good stir.

9. Stir in diced tomatoes and crushed tomatoes. When the mixture starts boiling, turn the heat to low heat and partially cover the pot.

10. Cook for about 30 minutes. Stir occasionally. Add kidney beans until the consistency you desire is achieved. Taste a little of the chili. Add some salt and other seasonings if desired.

11. Turn off the heat and let it sit covered for 5 minutes. You can serve it with low-carb cornbread or low-carb bread of your choice. You can also serve it with brown rice or cauliflower rice.

Ancho Chile Ground Beef Tacos

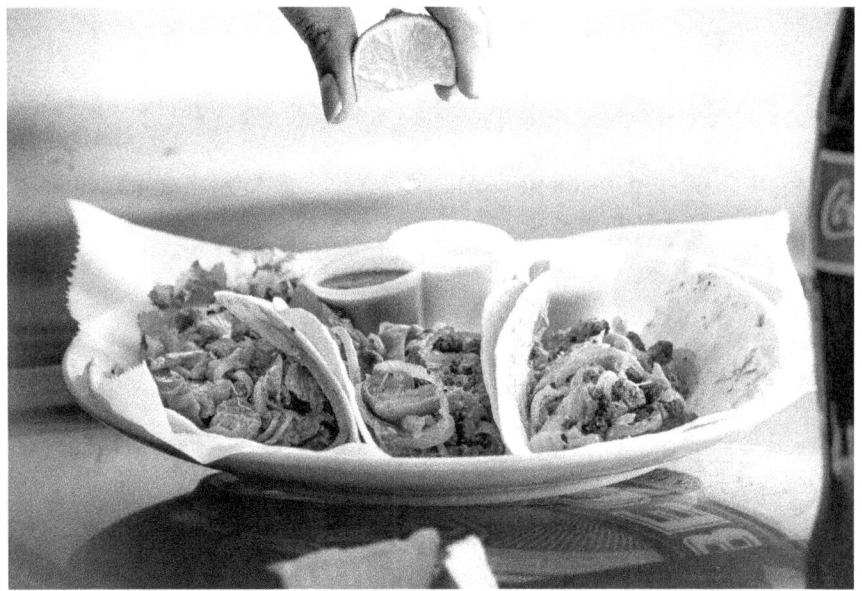

Serves: 2

Ingredients:

For taco seasoning:

- ½ tablespoon ancho chili powder
- ¼ teaspoon smoked paprika
- 1 teaspoon garlic powder
- ¼ teaspoon ground coriander
- ¼ teaspoon pepper or to taste
- ¾ teaspoon ground cumin
- ¾ teaspoon dried oregano

- ¾ teaspoon onion powder
- Sea salt to taste

For the beef tacos:

- 1 teaspoon cornstarch mixed with 2 – 3 tablespoons water
- 4 corn tortillas or taco shells or large lettuce leaves
- ½ pound lean ground beef (95% lean)
- ½ cup chopped romaine lettuce
- ¼ cup reduced-fat cheddar cheese
- 1 small onion, diced
- ½ red bell pepper, diced
- ½ yellow bell pepper, diced
- ½ can (from a 14 ounces can) diced tomatoes, drained
- ½ cup diced zucchini (optional)
- ½ cup canned or cooked black beans or kidney beans (optional)

Directions:

1. To make taco seasoning: Add chili powder, paprika, onion powder, salt, cumin, oregano, coriander, garlic powder, and pepper into a small bowl and stir.

2. Add beef into a skillet and cook for a couple of minutes over medium heat. As you stir, crumble the meat. Add onion, tomatoes, zucchini, and bell peppers and mix well.

Cook until the meat is brown. Discard extra cooked fat from the pan.

3. Add beans if using and stir. Add cornstarch mixture and taco seasoning. Stir constantly until thick. Let it cook for a couple of minutes. Stir often.

4. Serve meat filling over tortillas or lettuce leaves or tortillas. Scatter shredded lettuce and cheese on top and serve.

Cheesesteak Stuffed Peppers

Serves: 2

Ingredients:

- 2 bell peppers of any color, halved, deseeded, discard stem
- ½ large onion, sliced
- Salt to taste
- ¾ pound sirloin steak, thinly sliced
- 8 slices reduced fat provolone cheese
- ½ tablespoon vegetable oil
- 8 ounces cremini mushrooms, sliced
- Freshly ground pepper to taste
- 1 teaspoon Italian seasoning
- Chopped parsley to garnish

Directions:

1. Preheat the oven to 400° F.
2. Put the bell peppers in a baking dish, with the cut side facing up.
3. Put the baking sheet in the oven and set the timer for 20 to 30 minutes or until the peppers are tender. Set the oven to broil mode.
4. Pour oil into a skillet and let it heat over medium-high heat.

5. When the oil is hot, add mushrooms and onion and mix well. Season with salt and pepper. Cook until the vegetables are tender.

6. Stir in steak. Add some salt and pepper and cook for 3 minutes. Stir on and off.

7. Add Italian seasoning and mix well. Turn off the heat.

8. Place a slice of bell pepper on the bottom of each bell pepper half. Divide the meat mixture among the bell peppers. Place another slice of cheese in each bell pepper over the meat mixture.

9. Broil for 3 minutes or golden brown on top.

10. Sprinkle parsley on top and serve.

Beef Bourguignon Stew

Serves: 4

Ingredients:

- ¾ pound lean beef chuck, chopped into chunks
- 1 carrot, cut into ½-inch thick round slices
- 1 ½ tablespoons extra-virgin olive oil, divided
- ½ teaspoon dried oregano
- 2 sprigs thyme
- 1 clove garlic, minced
- ½ cup low-sodium beef stock
- 2 small onions, cut into large dice
- ¼ teaspoon pepper or to taste
- ½ pound russet potatoes, peeled, chopped into chunks
- 1 stalk celery, cut into thick slices
- A small sprig rosemary
- ½ pound button mushrooms, halved
- 2 small bay leaves
- 1 ½ tablespoons white-whole wheat flour or all-purpose flour
- 1 ½ cups pinot noir
- Kosher salt to taste

Directions:

1. Season the beef with salt and pepper. Sprinkle flour over the beef and toss well.

2. Pour half the oil into a pan and let it heat over medium-high heat. Add beef and cook until brown all over when the oil is hot. Stir occasionally.

3. Remove beef from the pan and place it in a bowl.

4. Pour a little of the wine and scrape the pot to remove any browned bits that may be stuck.

5. Stir in onion, mushrooms, rosemary, bay leaves, thyme, oregano, carrot, celery, and remaining oil and mix well.

6. After about 4 minutes, stir in garlic and cook for a few seconds until you get a nice aroma.

7. Stir in potatoes, salt, pepper, and beef. Pour stock and remaining wine. Give it a good stir. When the mixture starts boiling, turn down the heat to low heat and cook covered until meat and potatoes are cooked.

8. Serve hot with crusty whole-wheat bread or noodles or a salad or mashed cauliflower.

Thai Coconut Fish Curry

Serves: 4

Ingredients:

- ½ tablespoon olive oil or extra-virgin coconut oil
- 2 cloves garlic, minced
- ½ teaspoon finely grated lemon zest
- ¼ cup fish stock
- 1 tablespoon Thai green curry paste or more to taste
- 1 tablespoon fish sauce
- 1 cup canned, drained bamboo shoot strips
- ½ red bell pepper, deseeded, diced
- Toasted sesame seeds to garnish (optional)
- 1 onion, finely chopped
- ½ tablespoon minced ginger
- ½ cup vegetable stock
- 1 tablespoon fresh lime juice
- ½ cup light coconut milk
- 1 pound firm white fish, chopped into bite-size pieces
- 1 cup green peas, thawed if frozen
- ¼ cup finely chopped fresh cilantro
- Sea salt to taste

Directions:

1. Pour oil into a skillet and let it heat over medium heat. Add onions and cook until translucent. Stir in lime zest, ginger, and garlic.

2. Stir in vegetable stock. When the mixture starts boiling, turn down the heat to low heat. Cover the skillet and let it cook for about 15 minutes.

3. Add lime juice, curry paste, fish sauce, and coconut milk, and mix well.

4. Add fish, bamboo shoots, green peas, and bell pepper, and mix well.

5. Cover the skillet and continue cooking over medium-low heat until the fish is cooked.

6. Sprinkle cilantro and sesame seeds and serve over brown rice or cauliflower rice.

Grilled Shrimp Tacos with Cilantro Lime Coconut Cream Sauce

Serves: 4

Ingredients:

For the tacos:

- 1 ½ tablespoons olive oil, divided
- ½ teaspoon ground cumin
- ¼ teaspoon kosher salt
- 4 whole-wheat or corn tortillas (6 inches each)
- 1 clove garlic, minced
- ½ teaspoon chili powder or to taste
- 12 jumbo shrimp, peeled, deveined
- 1 cup shredded cabbage
- Chopped cilantro
- 1 tomato, chopped
- Chopped avocado

For cilantro lime coconut cream sauce:

- ¼ cup reduced-fat sour cream
- 1 teaspoon agave nectar
- ¼ teaspoon ground cumin
- Zest of ½ lime

- Juice of ½ lime
- 1 tablespoon light coconut milk
- 1/8 cup chopped fresh cilantro
- 1/8 teaspoon kosher salt or to taste

Directions:

1. To make the sauce: Add coconut milk, cilantro, lime juice, lime zest, salt, agave, cumin, and sour cream into a bowl and stir well.

2. Cover and refrigerate until use.

3. Add 1 tablespoon of oil, chili powder, cumin, salt, and garlic into a bowl and mix well.

4. Drop the shrimp into the bowl and turn it around to coat well.

5. Keep the bowl covered in the refrigerator for 30 – 60 minutes.

6. Set up your grill and preheat to medium heat.

7. Take 4 metal skewers and fix the shrimp on the skewers.

8. Place the skewers on the grill until the shrimp turn opaque, turning the skewers every 2 – 3 minutes.

9. Once grilled, take them out and keep it aside.

10. Brush the remaining oil over the tortillas and keep it on the grill. Cook for a minute and flip sides. Cook the other side for a minute. They should be slightly crisp but soft as well.

11. To assemble: Place 3 shrimp in the center of each tortilla. Divide the cabbage, cilantro, tomato, and avocado among the tortillas.

12. Drizzle sauce on top and serve.

Fish Taco Cabbage Bowls

Serves: 2

Ingredients:

- ¼ medium head red cabbage, thinly sliced
- 2 small white fish fillets, thawed in the refrigerator overnight if frozen
- 1 teaspoon fish rub
- ¼ teaspoon chili powder
- Guacamole to serve (optional but recommended)
- 2 teaspoons olive oil
- ½ teaspoon ground cumin
- ½ medium head green cabbage, thinly sliced
- ¼ cup thinly sliced green onions or more if desired

For dressing:

- 1 tablespoon fresh lime juice
- Salt to taste
- ¼ cup mayonnaise
- 1 teaspoon green Tabasco sauce or to taste

Directions:

1. Combine chili powder, fish rub, and cumin in a small bowl.

2. Dry the fish by patting with paper towels. Rub 1 teaspoon of oil on either side of the fish. Massage the rub mixture over the fish.

3. Set it aside for 15 – 20 minutes.

4. To make the dressing: Whisk together lime juice, salt, mayonnaise, and Tabasco sauce in a bowl.

5. Pour the remaining oil into a grill pan and let it heat over medium-high heat.

6. When the oil is hot, place the fish in the pan and cook for 4 minutes. Turn the fish over and cook the other side for 4 minutes or until the fish flakes easily when pierced with a fork. Turn off the heat and let the fish cool. Shred into smaller pieces using a pair of forks.

7. Place half the green onions, green, and red cabbage into a bowl and mix well.

8. Pour some of the dressing over the cabbage mixture and toss well.

9. To assemble: Divide the salad among 2 serving bowls. Drizzle remaining dressing on top.

10. Garnish with remaining green onions. Serve with guacamole if desired.

Angel Hair Pasta with Lemon Grilled Shrimp, Spinach, and Pine Nuts

Serves: 2 – 3

Ingredients:

- 4 ounces large shrimp, shelled, deveined
- Zest of ½ lemon
- Juice of ½ lemon
- ¼ teaspoon salt
- 1/8 cup nonfat Greek yogurt or mascarpone cheese
- 1/8 teaspoon freshly grated nutmeg
- 2 ½ cups fresh baby spinach
- 1/8 cup toasted pine nuts
- 4 ounces whole-grain angel hair pasta
- 1/8 cup shaved, reduced-fat parmesan cheese
- 1 clove garlic, minced
- ½ tablespoon butter, melted
- 1/8 teaspoon freshly ground pepper
- 1/8 cup fat-free half-and-half

Directions:

1. Set up your grill and preheat it to medium heat.
2. Dry the shrimp with paper towels and put them in a bowl.

3. Stir in lemon juice, garlic, pepper, lemon zest, salt, and melted butter. Cover the bowl and let it marinate for 30 minutes.

4. Fix the shrimp onto metal skewers and put it on the grill. After about 3 to 4 minutes, turn the skewers and cook for another 3 to 4 minutes or until the shrimp look cloudy.

5. Whisk together yogurt or mascarpone, nutmeg, and half-and-half in a bowl.

6. Cook the pasta following the directions given on the package of pasta. Drain the water but retain 3 – 4 tablespoons of the cooking water.

7. Add the cooked pasta into a pot. Add the yogurt sauce and stir well. Stir in the spinach and cook for a couple of minutes or until spinach wilts.

8. Add about a tablespoonful of the cooked pasta water and stir. If it is very thick, add more of the cooking water, a tablespoonful at a time and mix well each time.

9. When the spinach is tender, add salt and pepper to taste and turn off the heat.

10. Divide the pasta into 2 – 3 bowls. Divide equally the shrimp among the bowls.

11. Top with pine nuts and Parmesan cheese and serve.

Smoked Salmon Sushi Bowls

Serves: 2

Ingredients:

For the bowls:

- 1 cup cooked brown rice or cauliflower rice
- 6 ounces smoked salmon
- 2 small cucumbers, shaved into thin slices with a vegetable peeler
- ½ nori sheet, cut into strips
- Chopped, ripe avocado
- 1 small carrot, peeled, shaved into thin slices with a vegetable peeler
- Any other ingredients of your choice

For ginger sesame dressing:

- 1-inch piece of ginger, peeled, grated
- 2 teaspoons sesame oil
- ½ - 1 tablespoon honey
- 2 small cloves garlic, pressed
- Red pepper flakes to taste (optional)
- ½ tablespoon soy sauce or coconut aminos or tamari
- 1 ½ tablespoons rice vinegar

For spicy mayonnaise:

- 2 tablespoons sriracha sauce or more to taste
- 1 tablespoon mayonnaise
- ¼ teaspoon soy sauce or coconut aminos or tamari

Optional toppings:

- 1 teaspoon sesame seeds
- Pickled ginger
- 1 teaspoon wasabi paste
- 1 green onion, thinly sliced

Directions:

1. To make the dressing: Whisk together ginger, sesame oil, honey, garlic, red pepper flakes, soy sauce, and rice vinegar in a bowl.
2. Whisk together sriracha sauce, mayonnaise, and soy sauce and make the spicy mayonnaise.
3. Cover the bowl of dressing and spicy mayonnaise and keep them aside for a while for the flavors to infuse.
4. To assemble: Divide the rice into 2 serving bowls. Divide equally the smoked salmon, carrots, cucumber, and nori strips. Place any other desired toppings and optional toppings if desired.
5. Drizzle some ginger sesame dressing on top. Spoon the spicy mayonnaise on top of the bowls and serve.

Chapter Seven

Gastric Bypass Salad Recipes

Stage /Phase 2: Liquid and pureed diet (Generally 15 – 30 days after surgery but it can vary)

Classic Pureed Tuna Salad

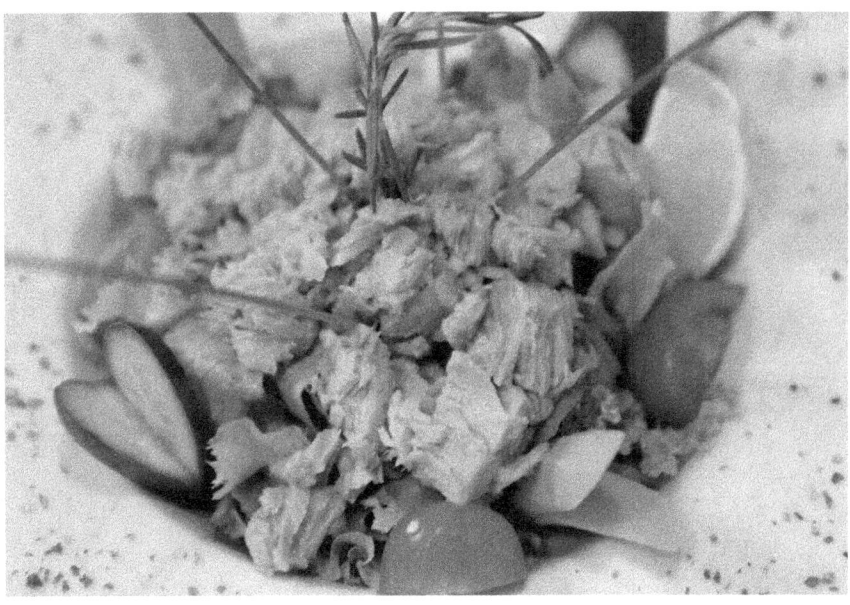

Serves: 1

Ingredients:

- ¼ can (from a 6 ounces can) tuna in water
- 2 teaspoons low-fat mayonnaise
- Salt to taste
- ½ teaspoon relish
- Pepper to taste
- 2 teaspoons nonfat plain Greek yogurt

Directions:

1. Add tuna and relish into the small blender jar. Blend until smooth.
2. Remove the mixture into a bowl. Add yogurt and tuna and mix well.
3. Add salt and pepper to taste if desired.
4. Divide into 2 bowls and serve.
5. For stage 3, in step 1, give short pulses until finely chopped. Continue with the remaining steps.
6. For stage 4, chop tuna into chunks. Add mayonnaise, relish, salt, pepper, and yogurt into a bowl and mix well. Add tuna and stir well.

Egg Salad

Serves: 2

Ingredients:

- 4 hard boiled eggs, peeled, chopped
- ¾ teaspoon celery salt
- A pinch mustard
- 4 – 5 tablespoons low-fat cottage cheese
- ¾ teaspoon onion powder
- Lettuce leaves (optional)

Directions:

1. Add eggs into a food processor. Pulse until eggs are chopped into small pieces.
2. Add celery salt, mustard, cottage cheese, and onion powder and process until smooth.
3. Divide into 2 bowls and serve one portion. Cover the other portion and place it in the refrigerator. Use it within 4 days.
4. This salad can be had in stages 3 and 4. For stage 3, the eggs in the salad should be finely chopped.
5. Crumble cottage cheese into a bowl. Add celery salt, mustard, and onion powder and mix well. Add some salt and pepper to taste. Add eggs and mix well.
6. For stage 4, chop the eggs into chunks and continue with step 5. Serve over lettuce leaves.

Stage /Phase 3: Soft diet (Generally between 5 – 12 weeks after surgery but it can vary)

Soft Crab Salad

Serves: 2

Ingredients:

- 4 ounces imitation crab, chopped into small pieces
- 1 scoop unflavored protein powder
- 1/8 teaspoon dried dill
- 2 tablespoons low-fat mayonnaise
- 1/8 teaspoon seafood seasoning

Directions:

1. Combine crab, mayonnaise, protein powder, seafood seasoning, and dill in a bowl.
2. Divide into 2 bowls and serve one portion. Cover the other portion and place it in the refrigerator. Use it within 4 days.

Chicken Salad

Serves: 2

Ingredients:

- ¼ cup plain nonfat Greek yogurt
- 2 tablespoons lime juice
- Freshly ground black pepper to taste
- ½ teaspoon ground cumin
- ½ avocado, peeled, pitted, cubed
- ¼ cup frozen corn, thawed (optional)
- Romaine lettuce to serve (optional)
- 1/8 cup low-fat sour cream
- 1 tablespoon chopped cilantro
- Sea salt to taste
- 1 boneless, skinless chicken breast, cooked, chopped
- ½ teaspoon chili powder
- ¼ cup cooked or canned black beans, drained, rinsed
- ½ red bell pepper, chopped

Directions:

1. To make the dressing: Combine sour cream, cilantro, salt, pepper, yogurt, lime juice, salt, chili powder, cumin, and pepper in a bowl.

2. Add chicken and beans into the food processor bowl and give short pulses until finely chopped. Transfer into a bowl. Add avocado and mix well. Add dressing and mix well.

3. For stage 4, do not chop the chicken and beans. Combine chicken, beans, avocado, bell pepper, and corn in a bowl. Add dressing and mix well.

4. Place lettuce leaves on a serving platter. Divide the salad equally and place it over lettuce leaves.

5. Serve.

Stage /Phase 4: Regular diet (Generally after 12 weeks after surgery but it can vary)

Taco Salad

Serves: 2 – 3

Ingredients:

- 1 teaspoon olive oil
- ½ teaspoon ground cumin
- ½ teaspoon chili powder
- 1 small onion, chopped
- ½ avocado, peeled, pitted chopped
- ½ head romaine lettuce, torn into bite-size pieces
- ½ pound extra-lean ground beef
- ½ teaspoon smoked paprika
- ½ teaspoon garlic powder
- ¼ cup low-fat Mexican cheese blend
- ½ cup halved cherry tomatoes

For the dressing:

- ½ tablespoon adobo sauce (from the can of chipotle chili in adobo sauce)
- Sea salt to taste
- 6 tablespoons low-fat sour cream

- ½ teaspoon lime juice
- Pepper to taste

Directions:

1. To make the dressing: Whisk together adobo sauce, salt, sour cream, lime juice, and pepper in a bowl. Cover and set it aside until the salad is ready.

2. Pour oil into a skillet and let it heat over medium-high heat. Add beef, cumin, chili powder, paprika, and garlic powder and mix well.

3. As you stir, crumble the meat into small pieces. Cook until the meat is brown.

4. Turn off the heat and let it cool for 10 minutes.

5. Transfer the meat into a bowl. Add avocado, lettuce, Mexican cheese, and tomatoes. Drizzle the dressing over the salad and stir well.

6. Serve.

Grilled Steak with Baby Arugula and Parmesan Salad

Serves: 2

Ingredients:

- ½ teaspoon chopped fresh thyme
- ¼ teaspoon freshly ground pepper or to taste
- 1 lemon, cut into 2 halves
- 2 cups loosely packed baby arugula
- 2 flat-iron steaks (4 ounces each)
- ½ ounce fresh parmesan cheese, shaved

For the dressing:

- ½ tablespoon extra-virgin olive oil
- ¼ teaspoon Dijon mustard
- ½ tablespoon chopped chives
- ½ tablespoon fresh lemon juice
- A pinch kosher salt
- ¼ teaspoon freshly ground black pepper or to taste

Directions:

1. Place a grill pan over medium-high heat on your stovetop.
2. Combine salt, pepper, and thyme in a small bowl and massage this mixture over the steak.

3. Place steak in the pan. After 4 minutes, flip sides. Cook for another 4 minutes or cook as per your preference.

4. Take the steak from the pan and place it on your cutting board. When it cools slightly, cut into thin slices across the grain.

5. Now place the lemon halves in the pan, with the skin side up. Cook for 3 minutes and turn off the heat.

6. To make the dressing: Whisk together oil, Dijon mustard, chives, lemon juice, salt, and pepper in a bowl.

7. Add arugula and mix well.

8. To assemble: Place 1 cup arugula on each of 2 serving plates. Place steak slices on each. Place a lemon half on each plate. Sprinkle a tablespoon of cheese on each.

9. Serve.

Strawberry Avocado Salad with Honey Glazed Grilled Salmon

Serves: 3

Ingredients:

For honey glaze:

- 1 tablespoon olive oil + extra to brush
- ½ tablespoon lemon juice
- Sea salt to taste
- ½ tablespoon honey
- ½ teaspoon liquid smoke

For the salad:

- 3 cups fresh spring lettuce mix
- ½ avocado, peeled, pitted, cut into cubes
- 2 ounces reduced-fat feta cheese, crumbled
- 2 wild Atlantic salmon fillets (4 ounces each), rinsed
- 5 – 6 strawberries, hulled, sliced
- 1/8 small red onion, thinly sliced
- 1/8 cup thinly sliced almonds, toasted

For honey balsamic dressing:

- Salt to taste
- 1 tablespoon balsamic vinegar

- ½ teaspoon Dijon mustard
- Freshly ground pepper to taste
- 2 tablespoons olive oil
- ½ tablespoon honey
- 1/8 teaspoon garlic powder

Directions:

1. To make honey glaze: Add oil, honey, lemon juice, salt, and liquid smoke into a bowl. Whisk well.
2. To make the honey balsamic dressing: Add salt, balsamic vinegar, mustard, pepper, olive oil, honey, and garlic powder into a small bowl. Whisk until well combined. Set aside until the salmon is grilled.
3. Set up your grill and preheat it to medium-high heat.
4. Dry the salmon by patting it with a clean towel. Brush the fillets with a little oil. Brush the grill grate with some oil.
5. Place salmon on the grill and close the lid. Grill for 4-5 minutes on each side.
6. Brush the honey glaze on the fillets and keep it aside.
7. Divide the spring mix lettuce between two plates. Divide the strawberries, onion, and avocados equally and place them over the lettuce. Top with cheese and almonds.
8. Pour dressing all over the salad. Place the grilled fillets on top. Drizzle the remaining glaze over the salmon if desired and serve.

Sardine Salad Niçoise

Serves: 2

Ingredients:

For the salad:

- 1 can Wild planet sardines in spring water
- 8 small black olives, pitted, halved
- 2 tablespoons red onion, thinly sliced
- 1 cup green beans, trimmed, cut into 1-inch pieces
- 4 cups mixed greens
- 8 grape tomatoes
- 1 large egg, hard-boiled, peeled, sliced

For the dressing:

- 2 tablespoons red wine vinegar
- 1 teaspoon Dijon mustard
- 3 tablespoons extra-virgin olive oil
- ¼ teaspoon freshly ground pepper or to taste
- ¼ teaspoon sea salt

Directions:

1. To make the dressing: Add vinegar and mustard into a bowl and whisk well. Pour oil in a thin stream, whisking

simultaneously. Whisk until it is slightly thick. Add salt and pepper to taste and mix well.

2. Place a nonstick pan over medium heat. Add beans and sauté for 2-3 minutes until crisp as well as tender. Turn off the heat.

3. Place 2 cups of greens on each of 2 serving plates. Divide equally and place sardines, egg, tomato, green beans, and onions over the greens.

4. Pour the dressing on top. Garnish with olives and serve.

Arugula Salad with Salmon, Avocado and Tomato

Serves: 2

Ingredients:

For the salad:

- 1 can salmon, drained, chopped into bite-sized pieces
- 3 cups baby arugula
- ½ medium avocado, peeled, pitted, cut into slices
- 2 tablespoons red onion, cut into thin slices
- 4 medium radishes, peeled, cut into thin slices
- 1 tomato, cut into ½-inch pieces

For the dressing:

- Sea salt to taste
- 1 tablespoon extra-virgin olive oil
- 1 tablespoon balsamic vinegar
- Freshly ground black pepper to taste
- ½ teaspoon honey

Directions:

1. To make the dressing: Add oil, vinegar, salt, honey, and pepper into a bowl and whisk well.

2. Place 1 ½ cups of arugula in each serving bowl. Layer with equal quantities of avocado, onion, radish, tomato, and salmon.

3. Pour the dressing over the salad and serve.

Herbed Shrimp with Tomato and Spinach Salad

Serves: 2

Ingredients:

- 1/8 cup chopped fresh flat-leaf parsley
- 1 tablespoon extra-virgin olive oil
- ¼ teaspoon sea salt
- ¼ teaspoon honey
- ½ cup halved heirloom grape tomatoes
- 2 cups baby spinach
- ¼ cup thinly sliced fennel bulb
- 1 ounce reduced-fat feta cheese, crumbled
- 1 tablespoon chopped fresh oregano
- 1 tablespoon red wine vinegar
- ¼ teaspoon freshly ground black pepper
- ½ pound large shrimp, peeled, deveined
- ¼ cup thinly sliced radicchio
- 1/8 cup torn mint leaves

Directions:

1. Spray a pan with cooking spray and place the pan over medium heat.

2. When the pan is hot, add shrimp and cook for a few minutes until the shrimp is pink and cooked. Add parsley and stir.

3. Turn off the heat.

4. To make the salad: Add salt, honey, red wine vinegar, honey, tomatoes, spinach, fennel, oregano, radicchio, pepper, and mint leaves into a large bowl and mix well.

5. Divide the salad into 2 bowls or plates. Top with feta cheese and shrimp and serve.

Mediterranean Tuna Salad

Serves: 2 – 3

Ingredients:

- 1 can (6 ounces) albacore tuna, drained
- ¼ cup sliced red grapes
- 1 tablespoon sliced kalamata olives
- 1 tablespoon chopped fresh basil
- 1 tablespoon lemon juice
- Sea salt to taste
- 1 large tomato, cut into slices
- 3 – 4 cups chopped dark greens of your choice
- Freshly ground pepper to taste
- ¼ cup sliced celery
- 1/8 cup thinly sliced red onion
- 1 tablespoon flat-leaf parsley
- ½ tablespoon chopped fresh oregano
- ½ tablespoon olive oil

Directions:

1. Add tuna, grapes, olives, basil, lemon juice, salt, pepper, celery, red onion, parsley, oregano, and olive oil into a bowl and toss well.

2. To serve: Divide the greens onto 2 serving plates. Place tomato slices over the greens.

3. Place tuna salad over the tomatoes and serve.

Grilled Shrimp Asian Salad with Thai Peanut Dressing

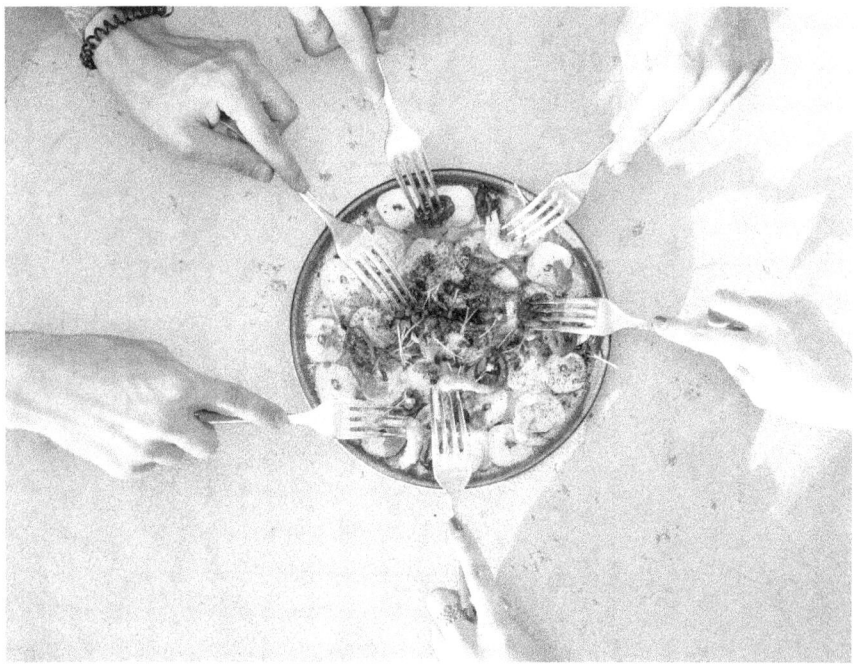

Serves: 2 – 3

Ingredients:

For Thai peanut dressing:

- 2 tablespoons olive oil or grapeseed oil
- 1 tablespoon unseasoned rice vinegar
- ½ tablespoon low-sodium soy sauce
- ½ tablespoon chopped fresh mint leaves
- 1 clove garlic, peeled, roughly chopped
- ½ teaspoon sea salt or to taste

- 1 tablespoon creamy peanut butter
- 1 tablespoon fresh lime juice
- ½ tablespoon honey
- ½ tablespoon chopped fresh ginger
- ½ teaspoon crushed red pepper flakes

For the salad:

- ½ pound large, fresh or frozen shrimp, peeled, deveined
- 2 ounces whole-wheat angel hair pasta
- ¼ cup thinly sliced cucumber
- 1/8 cup sliced green onions
- 1/8 cup chopped fresh basil
- 2 ounces baby spring-mix lettuce
- ¼ cup shredded carrots
- ¼ cup sliced red bell pepper
- ¼ cup sliced yellow bell pepper
- 1/8 cup chopped fresh cilantro

Directions:

1. To make Thai peanut dressing: Add peanut butter, lime juice, honey, ginger, red pepper flakes, oil, vinegar, soy sauce, mint leaves, garlic, and salt into the small blender jar and blend until smooth.

2. Place shrimp in a bowl. Add about 2 tablespoons of the peanut dressing and mix well.

3. Cover the bowl and let it sit for 30 – 60 minutes or until ready to use. If you are grilling it later than 60 minutes, place the bowl in the refrigerator.

4. Set up your grill and preheat to medium-high heat.

5. Fix the shrimp on skewers and put them on the grill. Cook for about 3 to 4 minutes. Turn the skewers over and cook the other side for 3 to 4 minutes.

6. Take out the skewers from the grill and set them aside to cool.

7. Meanwhile, cook the pasta following the directions given on the package of pasta.

8. To assemble: Spread lettuce leaves on a serving platter, and scatter carrots, basil, cilantro, cucumbers, and green onions over the top.

9. Place grilled shrimp on top. Pour remaining dressing on top and serve.

Chicken Avocado Caprese Salad

Serves: 3 – 4

Ingredients:

For the marinade/dressing:

- 2 tablespoons balsamic vinegar
- 1 teaspoon brown sugar
- ½ teaspoon dried basil
- ½ teaspoon sea salt
- 2 tablespoons olive oil
- ½ teaspoon minced garlic
- ½ teaspoon sea salt

For the salad:

- ½ pound boneless, skinless chicken breasts
- 2 ½ cups Romaine lettuce leaves, cut into bite-size pieces
- 1 cup halved cherry tomatoes
- ½ can (from a 14 ounces can) quartered artichoke hearts, drained
- Sea salt to taste
- Freshly ground pepper to taste
- ½ tablespoon olive oil
- ½ avocado, peeled, pitted, sliced

- ½ cup mini mozzarella cheese balls
- 1/8 cup thinly sliced basil

Directions:

1. To make marinade/dressing: Whisk together balsamic vinegar, brown sugar, basil, salt, olive oil, garlic, and sea salt in a bowl.

2. Add chicken and 2 tablespoons of the marinade into a Ziploc bag and fasten the bag. Turn the bag around a few times to coat the chicken well with the marinade.

3. Set aside for 30 minutes.

4. Pour ½ tablespoon of oil into a skillet and let it heat over medium-high heat. When the oil is hot, remove the chicken from the bag and place it in the skillet. The marinade from the bag is not needed, so discard it.

5. Cook the chicken for 6 – 7 minutes. Turn the chicken over and cook the other side for 6 – 7 minutes or until the chicken is cooked through inside.

6. Take out the chicken from the pan and place on your cutting board. When it cools for a while, cut into strips.

7. To assemble: Place the lettuce leaves on a serving platter. Scatter avocado over the lettuce, followed by artichoke hearts and tomatoes. Scatter mozzarella cheese balls all over and finally chicken.

8. Scatter basil on top. Pour the remaining marinade/dressing all over the salad.

9. Sprinkle salt and pepper to taste and serve.

Chicken Nachos Salad with Avocado Dressing

Serves: 2

Ingredients:

- 1 teaspoon Mexican chili powder
- 2 tablespoons extra-virgin olive oil
- 1 tablespoon grated pizza cheese
- 1 tablespoon finely chopped cilantro
- 3.5 ounces assorted cherry tomatoes, halved
- ¼ cup canned corn kernels
- ½ avocado, peeled, pitted, chopped
- ½ teaspoon finely grated lime zest
- 10.5 ounces small sweet potatoes, cut into wedges
- ½ tablespoon lime juice
- 8.8 ounces chicken breast
- ¼ small red onion, finely chopped
- 1 ounce mixed salad leaves
- ½ long green chili, thinly sliced

For dressing:

- ¼ ripe avocado, peeled, pitted, chopped
- ½ tablespoon chopped cilantro
- 1 tablespoon extra-virgin olive oil

- 1 tablespoon lime juice
- ½ tablespoon chopped mint leaves
- 1/8 cup buttermilk

Directions:

1. To make the dressing: Blend avocado, cilantro, oil, lime juice, mint leaves, and buttermilk in a blender until smooth. Pour into a bowl. Cover and set aside for a while for the flavors to meld.

2. Preheat the oven to 400° F.

3. Prepare a baking sheet by lining it with parchment paper.

4. Place sweet potatoes in a bowl. Drizzle 1 tablespoon oil over the sweet potatoes and toss well. Sprinkle chili powder, salt, lime zest, and pepper, and toss well.

5. Spread the sweet potatoes on the baking sheet and place them in the oven. Set the timer for 30 minutes or until the sweet potatoes are tender inside and brown outside.

6. Scatter cheese on top. Bake for a few minutes until the cheese melts.

7. Meanwhile, whisk together 1 tablespoon of oil, cilantro, and lime juice in a bowl. Add chicken and turn it around to coat.

8. Place a pan over medium-high heat and let it heat. Add chicken and cook until the underside is brown. Turn the

chicken over and cook the other side for about 4 minutes or until brown. Turn off the heat.

9. Remove chicken from the pan and place it on a cutting board. Tent the chicken loosely with foil. Cut into slices when it cools slightly.

10. To make the salad: Add tomatoes, corn, and onions into a bowl. Add salt and pepper to taste and stir until well combined.

11. Place mixed salad leaves on a serving platter. Place sweet potatoes, avocado, chicken, and tomato salad over the salad leaves, and drizzle the dressing over the top. Scatter green chili slices on top and serve.

Buttermilk Chicken with Chopped Salad

Serves: 3

Ingredients:

For the dressing/marinade:

- 1/3 cup low-fat buttermilk
- Juice of ½ lemon
- ½ tablespoon fresh thyme
- 1/8 teaspoon sea salt
- 1/8 teaspoon pepper

For chicken and salad:

- ¾ pound boneless, skinless chicken thighs, trimmed of fat, cut into ½-inch chunks
- ½ cucumber, chopped
- ½ cup halved red grapes
- ½ head Romaine lettuce or butter lettuce
- 1 small red onion, chopped

Directions:

1. Set up your grill and preheat it to medium-high heat.
2. To make the dressing: Add buttermilk, lemon zest, thyme, lemon juice, pepper, and salt into a bowl and stir until well

combined. Pour half of the dressing into another bowl and keep it aside.

3. Add chicken into the remaining dressing. Turn the chicken around in the dressing to coat it well. Let it marinate for 15 minutes.

4. Remove the chicken from the marinade and place it on the grill. This marinade is not required anymore so discard it.

5. Cook for about 10 minutes. Turn the chicken over and cook the other side for 10 minutes.

6. Place chicken on your cutting board. When it cools slightly, chop it into chunks.

7. To assemble: Combine lettuce, onion, cucumber, and grapes in a bowl.

8. Divide the salad among 3 plates. Top with chicken. Divide the dressing that was set aside into 3 small bowls. Place it on the side, next to the salad and serve.

Summer Strawberry and Chicken Salad with Sweet Thyme Dressing

Serves: 4 – 5

For the salad:

- 4 cups torn spring mix or spinach leaves
- 1 cup sliced fresh strawberries
- ¼ cup pecan halves
- 1/8 cup cooked, crumbled center-cut bacon
- 1 chicken breast, boneless, skinless
- Sea salt to taste
- ½ cup crumbled reduced-fat Gorgonzola cheese
- 1 tablespoon sugar or Splenda

For the sweet thyme dressing:

- 2 tablespoons red wine vinegar
- 1 teaspoon Dijon mustard
- ¼ teaspoon dried thyme or ¾ teaspoon finely chopped fresh thyme
- 1/8 teaspoon freshly ground pepper
- ¼ cup olive oil
- 1 ½ tablespoons agave nectar or Splenda
- 1 clove garlic, peeled, finely chopped
- ¼ teaspoon sea salt or to taste

Directions:

1. Set up your grill and preheat it to medium-high heat. Grease the grill grate with some oil.

2. Sprinkle salt and pepper over the chicken and place on the grill grate. Grill for about 8 – 10 minutes. Turn the chicken over and cook the other side for 8 – 10 minutes.

3. Place chicken on your cutting board. When it cools slightly, cut into slices.

4. To sugar-coat the pecans: Prepare a small baking sheet or plate by lining it with wax paper.

5. Add sugar and pecans into a small skillet. Place the skillet over medium-low heat.

6. Slowly the sugar will start to melt.

7. Keep stirring all the while. The melted sugar will coat the pecans. Turn off the heat when the sugar has completely melted and coats the pecans.

8. Transfer the pecans to the baking sheet and allow them to cool completely.

9. To assemble: Place lettuce in a serving bowl. Place chicken over the lettuce leaves followed by strawberries.

10. Scatter Gorgonzola cheese, sugar-coated pecans, and bacon crumbles on top and serve.

Red Quinoa, Couscous and Arugula Salad with Sweet Pimiento Dressing

Serves: 4

<u>For the salad:</u>

- 2 cups arugula
- 1 cup cooked red quinoa
- 1/8 cup sliced green onion
- 1/8 cup roasted pistachios (optional)
- 1 cup cooked Israeli couscous
- ¼ cup grated carrot
- 1/8 cup dried currants or blueberries

<u>For the dressing:</u>

- 1 clove garlic, peeled
- 1 tablespoon fresh lemon juice
- 1 tablespoon water
- 1/8 teaspoon sea salt or to taste
- 1/8 cup roasted red peppers
- ½ teaspoon grated lemon zest
- 1 tablespoon seasoned rice vinegar
- ½ teaspoon agave nectar
- 3 tablespoons olive oil

Marinade for lemon chicken (optional):

- 2 tablespoons fresh lemon juice
- ¼ teaspoon salt or to taste
- ½ pound trimmed, boneless, skinless chicken breasts
- ½ tablespoon Trader Joe's Seasoning Salute

Directions:

1. If you are using the chicken, prepare it first: Put the chicken in a Ziploc bag.

2. Add lemon juice, salt, and Trader Joe's Seasoning Salute and seal the bag.

3. Turn the bag around a few times so that chicken is well coated with the marinade.

4. Place the bag in the refrigerator for 4 – 8 hours.

5. Set up your grill and preheat it to medium-high heat. Grease the grill grate with some oil.

6. Take out the chicken from the bag and place it on the grill grate. Grill for about 8 – 10 minutes. Turn the chicken over and cook the other side for 8 – 10 minutes. The marinade is no longer required.

7. Place chicken on your cutting board. When it cools slightly, cut into slices.

8. To make the dressing: Add garlic, lemon juice, water, salt, roasted red pepper, lemon zest, vinegar, agave nectar, and oil into a blender and blend until smooth.

9. Cook the quinoa and couscous following the directions on the package.

10. Add arugula, quinoa, green onion, pistachios, couscous, carrot, and currants into a bowl and mix well.

11. You can use the blended dressing or strain the dressing and use the strained dressing. Discard the solids if straining.

12. Pour dressing over the salad. Toss well. Divide the salad equally and place it on serving plates. Top with chicken slices and serve.

Summer Salad with Buttermilk Vinaigrette

Serves: 2

Ingredients:

For dressing:

- 1/8 cup buttermilk
- ¼ teaspoon sea salt
- 1 tablespoon olive oil
- 1 tablespoon chopped fresh dill
- ½ tablespoon chopped oregano
- 1 tablespoon white wine vinegar
- 1/8 teaspoon pepper
- ½ clove garlic, minced
- 1 tablespoon finely chopped chives
- ½ tablespoons roughly chopped tarragon

For the salad:

- ½ shallot, very thinly sliced
- 1 ear raw, fresh sweet corn, remove the kernels
- ½ cup halved cherry tomatoes
- 1 tablespoon chopped oregano
- 1 tablespoon finely chopped fresh dill
- Sea salt to taste

- ½ medium English cucumber, finely diced
- ½ red bell pepper, deseeded, finely diced
- 1 tablespoon chopped tarragon
- 1 tablespoon finely chopped fresh chives

Directions:

1. To make the dressing: Blend buttermilk, salt, oil, dill, oregano, vinegar, garlic, chives, and tarragon in the small blender. Blend until well incorporated.

2. Transfer the dressing into a bowl and chill for at least 4 hours for the flavors to meld.

3. To make the salad: Add corn kernels, cherry tomatoes, shallot, cucumber, bell pepper, oregano, dill, tarragon, and chives into a bowl and toss well.

4. Pour dressing over the salad just before serving. Toss well and serve.

Rainbow Salad with Za'atar Yogurt Dressing

Serves: 1

Ingredients:

For the salad:

- ¼ cup diced carrots
- ¼ cup shredded red cabbage
- ¼ cup diced sweet bell pepper of any color
- ¼ cup diced cucumber
- ¼ cup diced beets
- ¼ cup cooked or canned chickpeas or any beans of your choice
- ½ cup chopped salad leaves
- 4 – 5 baby tomatoes, halved
- ½ cup diced avocado
- 1 small onion, sliced
- ¼ cup cubed tofu
- 4 – 5 fresh mint leaves, torn

For the dressing:

- ½ tablespoon lemon juice
- ¼ teaspoon ground black pepper
- 1/8 teaspoon kosher salt

- ½ tablespoon za'atar spice blend
- ½ cup plain nonfat Greek yogurt

Directions:

1. You can serve this salad in a glass bowl or on a plate. You can layer the ingredients or mix them up together. Either way, it looks appealing.

2. You can use cooked or raw beets; the choice is yours. If you want to use cooked beets, you can either steam them or roast them.

3. Place salad leaves in a bowl.

4. Layer carrots, cabbage, bell pepper, cucumber, beets, chickpeas, tomatoes, avocado, tofu, and onion in any colorful manner you desire or mix them up. Sprinkle mint leaves on top

5. Cover and chill until use.

6. To make the dressing: Whisk together lemon juice, yogurt, pepper, salt, and za'atar spice blend in a bowl.

7. Cover and chill until ready to use.

8. Pour dressing over the salad just before serving.

Cucumber, Corn, Black Bean, and Avocado Salad

Serves: 2

Ingredients:

- ½ English cucumber, peeled, diced
- 2/3 cup corn kernels, fresh or frozen
- ½ cup assorted cherry tomatoes
- Juice of ½ lime
- Sea salt to taste
- ½ can (from a 15 ounces can) black beans, rinsed, drained
- ½ red bell pepper, diced
- ¼ cup packed chopped fresh cilantro
- Pepper to taste
- ½ ripe avocado, peeled, pitted, diced

Directions:

1. Add black beans, cucumber, corn, cherry tomatoes, red pepper, and cilantro into a bowl and toss well.
2. Add lime juice, salt, pepper, and avocado and mix well.
3. Serve.

Thai Quinoa Salad

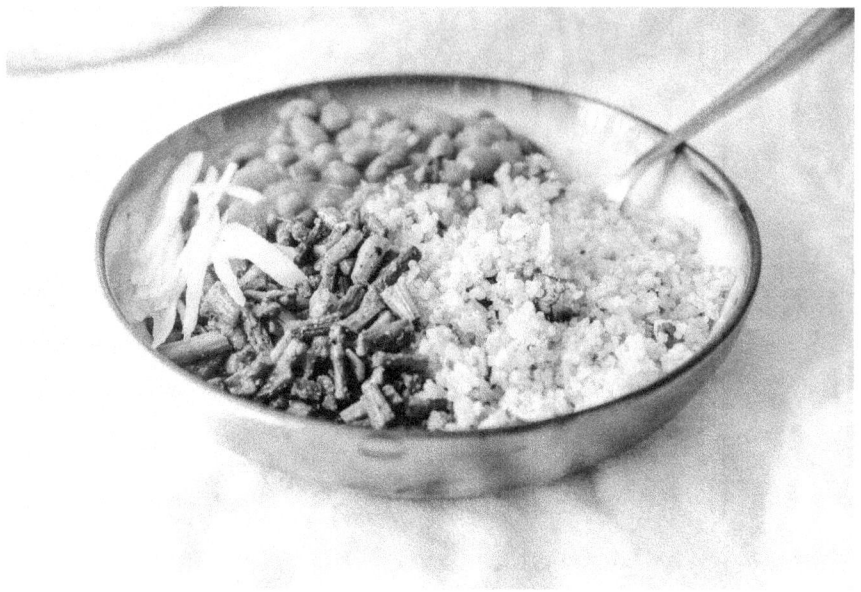

Serves: 1

For dressing:

- ½ tablespoon sesame seeds
- ½ teaspoon fresh lemon juice
- 1 teaspoon tamari
- ½ date, pitted
- ¼ teaspoon toasted sesame oil
- ½ teaspoon garlic, chopped
- 1 ½ teaspoons apple cider vinegar
- 2 tablespoons tahini

- ¼ teaspoon sea salt or to taste
- Water, as required

For salad:

- ½ cup quinoa, rinsed
- ½ tomato, sliced
- 1 small red onion, chopped
- 1 cup arugula

Directions:

1. To make the dressing: Add a little water, sesame seeds, lemon juice, tamari, dates, sesame oil, garlic, vinegar, tahini, and salt into a blender and blend until smooth. Check for the consistency of the dressing and add more water if required.

2. Pour 1-inch of water into a saucepan and let it heat over medium heat. Place a steamer basket in it and place quinoa in it. Steam for 15-20 minutes until tender.

3. Fluff the quinoa grains with a fork and spread them on a plate to cool.

4. Add quinoa, tomato, onion, and arugula into a bowl and toss well. Pour dressing on top. Mix well and serve.

Southwestern Salad with Black Beans

Serves: 2

Ingredients:

- 1 ripe avocado, peeled, pitted, chopped
- 1 cup nonfat plain yogurt
- 2 cloves garlic, quartered
- 1 teaspoon sugar or Splenda
- 6 cups mixed greens
- 1 cup corn kernels, fresh or frozen, thaw if frozen
- 1 ½ cups fresh cilantro
- 4 scallions, chopped
- 2 tablespoons lime juice
- 1 teaspoon salt
- 1 cup cooked or canned black beans
- 1 cup grape tomatoes

Directions:

1. Blend avocado, yogurt, lime juice, sugar, salt, cilantro, garlic and scallions in a blender until smooth.

2. Put the mixed greens into a bowl. Add 4 tablespoons of the dressing and mix well.

3. Place black beans, tomatoes and corn over the greens.

4. Drizzle the remaining dressing over it. You can add all of the dressing or use as much as required and store the remaining dressing in an airtight container in the refrigerator. Use it within 3 days

Spiralized Apple Salad

Serves: 2

Ingredients:

- ½ large red apple (like honey crisp or gala or pink lady), cored
- ½ large orange, peeled, separated into segments
- ½ large Granny Smith apple
- 3 tablespoons pecans
- ½ tablespoon sunflower seeds
- 1 ounce sharp white cheddar cheese, cut into ¼-inch cubes
- 1/8 cup dried, chopped unsweetened cranberries
- ½ teaspoon chia seeds (optional)

For the dressing:

- 3 tablespoons olive oil
- 1 tablespoon orange juice
- 1/8 teaspoon kosher salt
- 1 tablespoon lemon juice
- 1 tablespoon grated lemon zest
- ½ tablespoon grated orange zest
- ¾ teaspoon honey or maple syrup
- Pepper to taste

Directions:

1. To make the dressing: Blend oil, orange juice, salt, lemon juice, lemon zest, orange zest, maple syrup, and pepper in the small blender jar until smooth. You can also mix them in a bowl.

2. Make noodles of the apples using a spiralizer or julienne peeler.

3. Place apple noodles, orange, cranberries, pecans, cheese, sunflower seeds, and chia seeds in a bowl and toss well.

4. Pour dressing over the salad. Toss well and serve.

Three Bean Mediterranean Salad

Serves: 2 – 3

Ingredients:

For the salad:

- 4 ounces green beans, trimmed, cut into 2-inch pieces
- ½ can (from a 15 ounces can) red kidney beans, rinsed, drained
- ½ red or green bell pepper, diced
- ½ can (from a 15 ounces can) chickpeas, rinsed, drained
- ½ English cucumber, sliced
- 1 small red onion, sliced
- ¼ cup loosely packed mint leaves, chopped
- ¼ cup loosely packed parsley leaves, chopped
- 1/8 cup loosely packed fresh basil leaves, chopped
- 1/8 cup capers (optional)
- ¼ cup reduced-fat feta cheese chunks (optional)

For the dressing:

- 1 ½ tablespoons red or white wine vinegar
- ½ tablespoon Dijon mustard
- Freshly ground pepper to taste
- 1/8 teaspoon smoked paprika

- ½ clove garlic, minced
- Juice of ½ lemon
- ¼ teaspoon sea salt or to taste
- ½ teaspoon honey, agave nectar or Splenda
- 1 tablespoon finely diced red onion
- ¼ cup olive oil

Directions:

1. Cook green beans in a microwave-safe bowl in the microwave for 2 minutes.

2. Have a bowl of ice water ready on your countertop. Once the beans are cooked, put them into a bowl of ice water.

3. Let it cool for 5 minutes. Drain in a colander.

4. In a bowl, combine green beans, kidney beans, chickpeas, bell pepper, basil, mint, parsley, and cucumber.

5. To make the dressing: Blend together vinegar, mustard, pepper, paprika, garlic, lemon juice, salt, honey, onion, and oil in a blender until smooth.

6. Pour the dressing over the salad. Toss well and serve.

Winter Green Salad with Pomegranate Dressing

Serves: 2 – 3

Ingredients:

For the salad:

- 1 cup spring salad mix
- 1 stalk celery, sliced
- ½ pear, cored, peel if desired, chopped
- 1/8 cup chopped pecans
- 1 cup shaved Brussels sprouts
- 1 small red onion, thinly sliced
- 1/8 cup dried cranberries, unsweetened

For the dressing:

- 1/8 cup apple cider vinegar
- ½ teaspoon Dijon mustard
- 3 tablespoons olive oil
- ¼ cup pomegranate juice
- ½ tablespoon sugar or Splenda
- 1/8 teaspoon garlic powder
- 1/8 teaspoon sea salt
- 1/8 teaspoon freshly ground black pepper

Directions:

1. To make the dressing: Add pomegranate juice, apple cider vinegar, sugar, Dijon mustard, garlic powder, salt, pepper, and oil into a small jar.

2. Fasten the lid and shake the jar vigorously for a few seconds until well combined.

3. To make the salad: Add celery, spring mix, onion, and Brussels sprouts into a bowl and toss well.

4. Distribute equally the salad among 2 – 3 serving plates. Distribute pear slices, pecans, and cranberries equally over the salad.

5. Drizzle the dressing over the salad and serve.

Summer Salad with Creamy Italian Dressing

Serves: 2 – 3

Ingredients:

- 3 cups spring mix salad greens
- ½ cup cauliflower florets
- ½ cup diced, reduced-fat Swiss cheese
- 1/8 cup dried blueberries, unsweetened
- ½ cup broccoli florets
- ½ cup halved, assorted cherry tomatoes
- 1 small red onion, sliced
- 3 slices center-cut bacon, cooked, crumbled

For creamy Italian dressing:

- ¼ cup plain nonfat Greek yogurt
- 1/8 cup white wine vinegar
- 1 tablespoon agave nectar or swerve or Splenda to taste
- ¼ teaspoon Italian seasoning
- 1/8 teaspoon freshly ground black pepper
- 1/8 cup low-fat mayonnaise
- 1 tablespoon fresh lemon juice
- ¼ teaspoon garlic powder
- ¼ teaspoon sea salt
- 1/8 teaspoons dried dill

Directions:

1. To make the dressing: Add yogurt, white wine vinegar, agave nectar, Italian seasoning, pepper, mayonnaise, lemon juice, garlic powder, sea salt, and dill into a blender and blend until smooth.

2. To make the salad: Add cauliflower and broccoli into a microwave-safe bowl and cook on High for 2 – 3 minutes or until crisp as well as tender. Make sure you do not overcook.

3. Drain in a colander. Immerse the cauliflower and broccoli in a bowl of chilled water for a few minutes until it cools down.

4. Place tomatoes, onion, salad greens, blueberries, cauliflower, broccoli, and bacon into a bowl and toss well.

5. Pour the dressing over the salad. Toss well and serve.

Watermelon Tomato Salad

Serves: 1 – 2

Ingredients:

For the dressing:

- 2 teaspoons tamari or soy sauce
- 1 ½ teaspoons rice vinegar
- ¼ inch fresh ginger, peeled, minced
- 1 ½ teaspoons fresh lime juice
- ½ clove garlic, minced
- Sea salt to taste (optional)

For the salad:

- 2 heirloom tomatoes, cut into wedges
- ½ jalapeño, thinly sliced
- 4 cashews, quartered, toasted
- Lime wedges to serve
- 4 cups watermelon chunks
- Pepper to taste
- 1 ½ tablespoons chopped Thai basil or normal basil to garnish
- 1/3 avocado, peeled, pitted, diced
- Sea salt to taste

Directions:

1. Prepare the dressing by whisking together lime juice, ginger, garlic, vinegar and tamari in a bowl.

2. Add watermelon, tomatoes, and jalapeños into 1 – 2 shallow bowls.

3. Pour dressing on top. Sprinkle salt and pepper to taste. Place the avocado, lime wedges, cashews, and basil on top.

4. Serve.

Orzo Salad

Serves: 3

Ingredients:

- ¾ cup whole-grain orzo pasta
- ½ tablespoon red wine vinegar
- ¼ teaspoon dried oregano
- 1 Persian cucumber, halved lengthwise, cut into ¼ inch thick slices crosswise
- ½ cup cooked or canned chickpeas, rinsed, drained
- 1 small red onion, thinly sliced
- ½ cup fresh basil or mint leaves (you can use a mixture of both)
- ½ tablespoon fresh lemon juice
- 1/8 teaspoon sea salt
- 1 cup halved cherry tomatoes
- 2 ounces reduced-fat feta cheese, cut into ¼-inch cubes
- ¼ cup pitted kalamata olives
- Freshly ground pepper to taste
- Olive oil to drizzle

For the dressing:

- 2 tablespoons extra-virgin olive oil
- ½ clove garlic, minced

- 1/8 teaspoon Dijon mustard or to taste
- Freshly ground pepper to taste
- 1 ½ tablespoons red wine vinegar
- ¼ teaspoon dried oregano + extra to garnish
- 1/8 teaspoon sea salt

Directions:

1. To make the dressing: Add vinegar, oregano, salt, olive oil, garlic, mustard, and pepper into a bowl and whisk well. Cover and set aside until the salad is ready.

2. Cook pasta following the directions given on the package of pasta.

3. Pour a little olive oil over the pasta and toss well. Let it cool completely. You can also have a warm salad if desired.

4. Add orzo, tomatoes, feta, olives, red onion, chickpeas, and cucumber into a bowl and toss well.

5. Pour dressing over the salad. Toss well and serve.

Conclusion

I want to thank you once again for choosing this book. I hope it proved to be an enjoyable and informative read.

Undergoing a gastric bypass diet will change your life. The primary focus after the surgery must be on recovery and internal healing while retaining the different benefits it offers. One of the most important aspects that you must focus on during this stage is the diet you follow. This diet is known as the gastric bypass diet and is designed to promote the healing of your stomach and ensure that your body slowly gets accustomed to eating solid foods as you did before. This diet prescribes a four-stage approach for recovery and healing. The dietary recommendations usually vary from one individual to another, but you will still need to work your way through these four stages. You will consume only fluids during the first stage, while pureed foods are introduced in the second stage. The third and fourth stages reintroduce soft foods and solid foods, respectively. Moving from the first to the fourth stage can take at least six weeks and even longer, depending on your recovery. Just because you are concentrating on recovery doesn't mean you need to consume boring meals. You can still eat flavorful and wholesome meals, provided you get a little creative with the ingredients used. This is where this book steps into the picture.

So, what are you waiting for? It is never too late to regain control over your health and improve it. All the different suggestions and tips, along with nutritional requirements for a prescribed gastric diet, were presented in this book. You were also introduced to a plethora of delicious, healthy, and simple gastric bypass diet-friendly recipes. Forget spending hours in the kitchen cooking meals during recovery. Instead, you simply need to select the recipes from this book that strike your fancy, gather the required ingredients, and follow the simple steps mentioned in this book. These are the only steps you need to follow. A little creativity and an open mindset go a long way when it comes to following a healthy diet that is flavorful and holds them.

Thank you for buying and reading/listening to our book. If you found this book useful/helpful please take a few minutes and leave a review on Amazon.com or Audible.com (if you bought the audio version).

Resources

A guide to eating after gastric bypass surgery. (2018). Mayo Clinic.

Dietary Guidelines After Bariatric Surgery. (2019, March 14). Ucsfhealth.org; UCSF Health.

What to Eat and Drink Before and After Your Gastric Bypass Surgery. (2020, August 24). Healthline.

www.ingramcontent.com/pod-product-compliance
Lightning Source LLC
Chambersburg PA
CBHW071353210526
45465CB00001B/82